Guruji BKS Iyengar

and his institute in the '70s

Foreword by Geeta S Iyengar

Compiled by Julia Pedersen

Photographs by Georg and Julia Pedersen

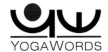

YOGAWORDS

Guruji BKS Iyengar and his institute in the '70s

First published in the UK by YogaWords, an imprint of Pinter & Martin Ltd 2020

ISBN 978-1-906756-65-9

Also available as an ebook

Design and photo retouching by Priyadarshi Sharma

British Library Cataloguing-in-Publication Data
A catalogue record for this book is available from the British Library

Printed in the EU by Hussar

This book has been printed on paper that is sourced and harvested from sustainable forests and is FSC accredited

YogaWords c/o Pinter & Martin Ltd
6 Effra Parade
London SW2 1PS

yogawords.com

Contents

Contributors

AC Alan Cameron, UK
16, 23, 25, 27, 61, 188

AD Ayesha Devi, India
10, 30, 34, 47, 51

AJ Abhay Javakhedkar, India
52, 122, 173, 177

BC Bobby Clennell, USA
16, 33, 63, 93, 189

BM Birjoo Mehta, India
41, 42, 44, 63, 75, 81, 162

CC Caroline Coggins, Australia
28, 65, 114

CD Colle Dastur, India
86, 87, 121

EH Evlaleah Howard, USA
155, 189

FAR Firooza Ali Razvi, India
12, 30, 35, 44, 58, 75, 85, 109, 119, 121, 125, 133, 171, 191

FB Faeq Biria, France
50, 189

FJP Father Joe Pereira, India
75, 166, 177, 188

GG Gabriella Giubilaro, Italy
28, 85, 98, 153

JB Jawahar Bangera, India
52, 83, 177

JP Julia Pedersen, Australia
25, 36, 63, 66, 85, 95, 96, 103, 126, 141, 146, 150

JW Joan White, USA
10, 54, 78, 83, 96, 164, 168

KP Kay Parry, Australia
137, 189

KW Karen Wilde, Australia
33

LS Lois Steinberg, USA
141, 149, 181, 191

ND Neeta Datta, India
85, 98

NK Navaz Kamdin, India
18, 21, 54, 119

NY Naoko Yagyu, Japan
79

PD Peter Davies, Australia
153

PL Pixie Lillas, Australia
12, 14, 16, 18, 42, 47, 48, 57, 68, 77, 113, 191

PR Pandurang Rao, India
179

PS Peter Scott, Australia
90

PT Peter Thompson, Australia
36

PW Patricia Walden, USA
30, 39, 48, 101, 156

RAW Richard Agar Ward, UK
39, 61

RM Rajvi Mehta, India
72, 104, 122, 131, 163, 164, 188

RN Rajlaxmi Nidmarti, India
41, 137

SC Swati Chanchani, India
23, 119, 135, 191

SQ Stephanie Quirk, Australia
88, 109, 124, 143, 145, 182

UD Usha Devi, India
161

VD Vinod Dalal, India
14, 65, 81, 158, 159

ZZ Zubin Zarthoshtimanesh, India
83, 167

NOTE ON CONTRIBUTORS' NAMES: The first time a contributor is listed in the book, both their initials and name are printed. In all subsequent listings, they are named only by their initials.

Introduction
How this book came about

I first started going to study with Guruji, Geetaji and Prashantji at the Ramamani Iyengar Memorial Yoga Institute (RIMYI) in 1976. It was an exciting time to be there, as the Institute had just opened the year before. Small groups of students came from all over the world to join the local people in the general classes as well as to take part in special intensives.

A couple of years later my husband Georg Pedersen was with me attending classes. He asked Guruji for permission to take some photos as he was a keen amateur photographer at that time. A few photos were also taken by me, and in total there were well over 200 black and white negatives sitting in a folder in my filing cabinet since then. It wasn't until Guruji died and we were missing him that I finally got the old negatives scanned. Many people have seen these photos now and have told me what a great insight it gives them into what it was like to be there then. I was encouraged to put together a book so that everyone can have access to them.

In talking to some of the old students who were there at the time, I felt that adding their stories as a narrative would help to give at least an inkling of what it was like to be there then. We were incredibly fortunate to be there at that special time and we would like to share it with you. It is my hope that this book can give you a glimpse into that precious and inspiring time.

All royalties from the book go to RIMYI to further Iyengar yoga in India.

Julia Pedersen
Sydney, Australia, 2020

To Guruji, our beloved teacher,
and to the whole Iyengar family
who have given us all so much.

Foreword

Guruji BKS Iyengar would have been 100 on 14th December 2018. He started teaching in 1936 and was teaching up to the last breath. One will not believe, if I say that just 15 days before his demise he was sitting on the balcony facing the hall and saw someone doing *Ardha Chandrasana* wrongly near the grills and pointed out the mistake asking the teacher to correct. The person was happy and saluted Guruji from the hall. Nothing missed his sharp penetrative eyes.

Julia Pedersen, my great friend, has done a wonderful job of joining the photographs with the reflections of the students from the '70s or even earlier from every corner of the world. Many of the pupils have not seen him when he was dynamic, fast and swift in his movements. His eyes were shining and the arms were ever-ready to help. He used to move from one pupil to another in a fraction of a second and touch the pupil exactly where the touch was needed.

True that photos cannot talk to you, but Julia has done it. The picture not only informs you, but talks to you as lively as Guruji was. Such an active, positive and dynamic personality was our 'Guruji'. He is our divine guide who sends the messages when we are fully awake or in deep sleep. We cannot forget him even in our dreams. Many people have experienced it.

I request you all to treasure this book in your heart. Do not just read or see the pictures, but feel Guruji's divine presence and nearness. The book will talk to you. The book will make you see beyond. The book will take you towards Guruji. It will inspire you spiritually to be on the path of pure yoga which Guruji gave us with sanity, sanctity and Divinity.

Geeta S Iyengar
RIMYI, Pune, December 2018

The Classes

I can still remember the sheer energy, the whole dynamism of those classes with him. His courage to make us do the things he did. He was so sure of his art and you felt so safe in his hands, no matter what he did. He gave you total confidence even in the most difficult things.

AD (Ayesha Devi)

He created an intense atmosphere that demanded every moment of my attention and focus. We had no time to think about anything other than what he was saying and wanting us to do. It was scary yet exhilarating at the same time. I was amazed at his ability to communicate what he wanted even when he didn't have the language. He was mercurial in his ability to notice what was happening and to change how he was expressing himself until all could understand. He was fascinating. He was the best teacher I had ever experienced in his ability to communicate with his class. I was hooked.

JW (Joan White)

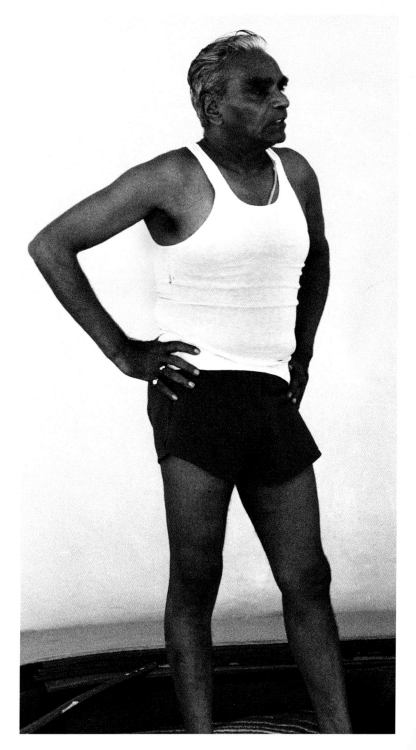

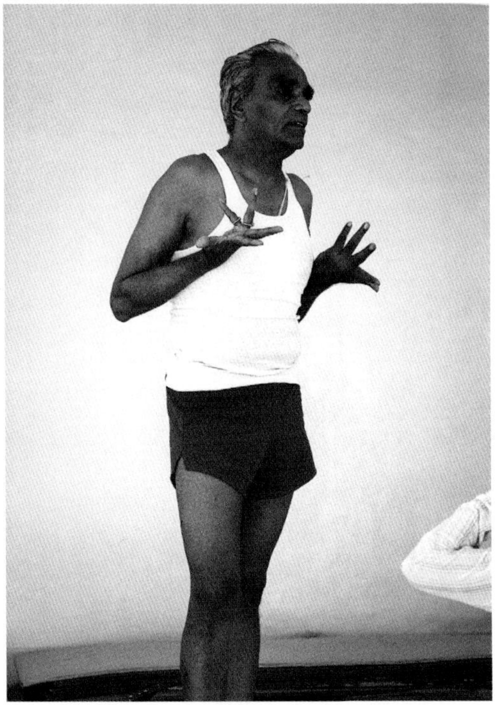
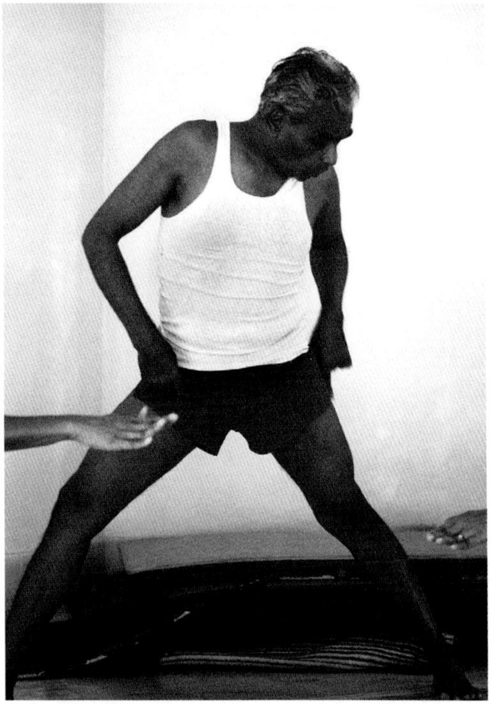
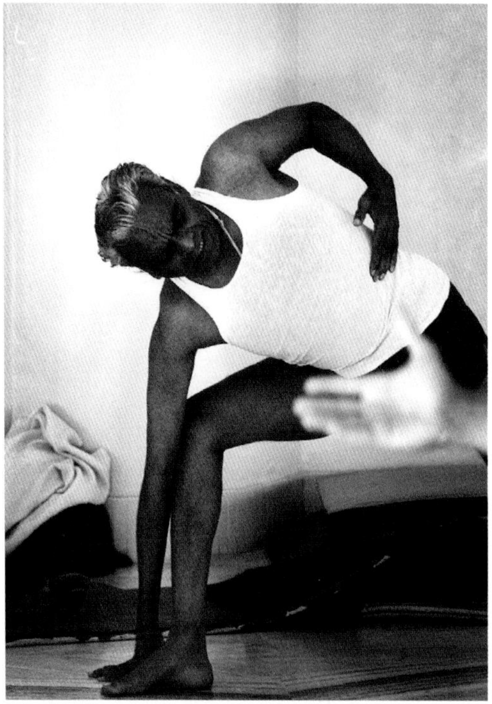
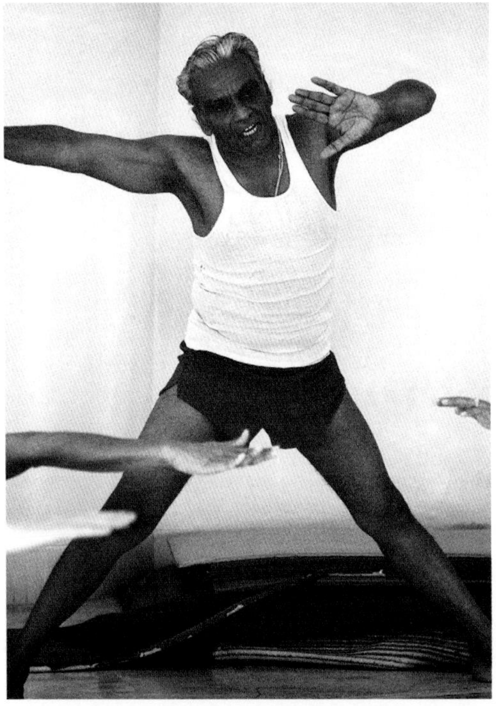
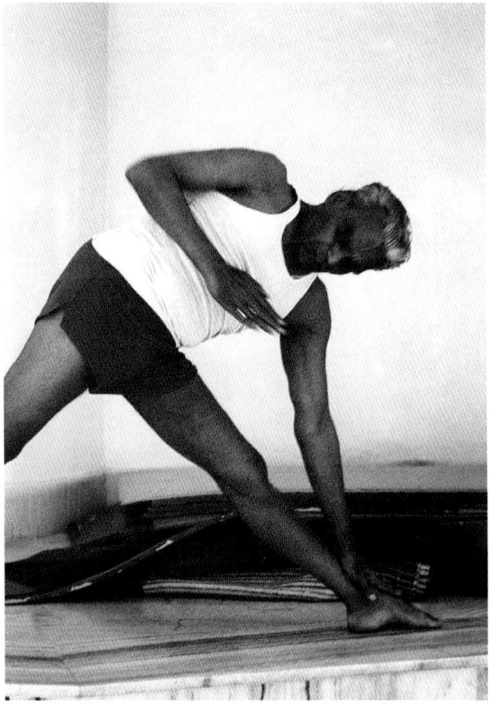
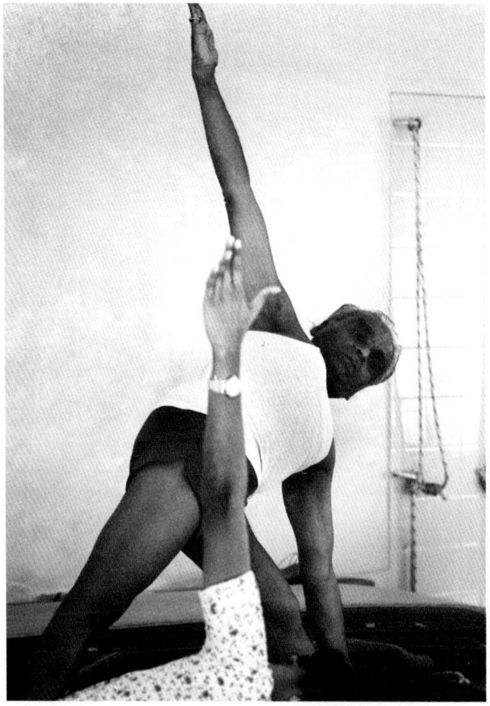

Every day we would walk down Fergusson College Road from our hotels and then turn down Hare Krishna Mandir Road. We would be in a group, chatting and laughing about nothing in particular. The last 200 metres we would all invariably fall silent, with a mixture of nerves and excitement taking over. What would happen today? We would distractedly try to fill in the time before class started with a few warm up poses, and suddenly we would hear a sharp *"UTTANASANA"* from the entrance to the hall. Guruji had appeared out of nowhere, and an electric bolt would go through us all. We then surrendered entirely to the class, whatever it contained.

PL (Pixie Lillas)

He was always full of surprises. Guruji never started the class with 'the usual.' What happened was that we were all there 100%. He was about 60 years old and I was just around 20—I couldn't get over the fact that he appeared younger and more energetic than us at that age of 20. It was unbelievable that this man could be nearing 60. Most people are retired at that age. His energy and his very presence were very magnetic, very electrifying.

FAR (Firooza Ali Razvi)

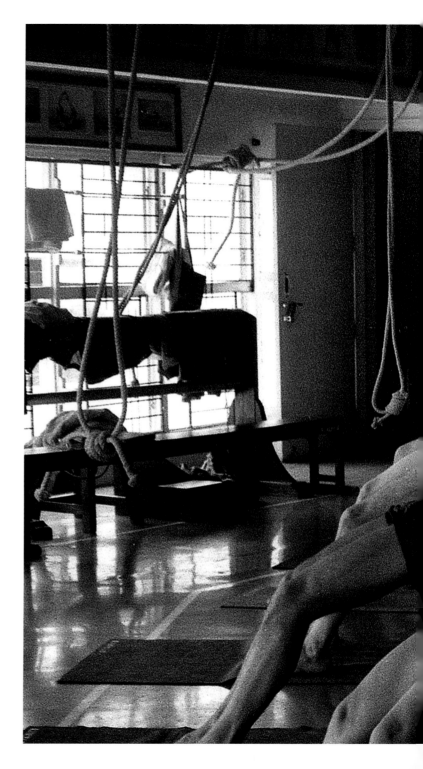

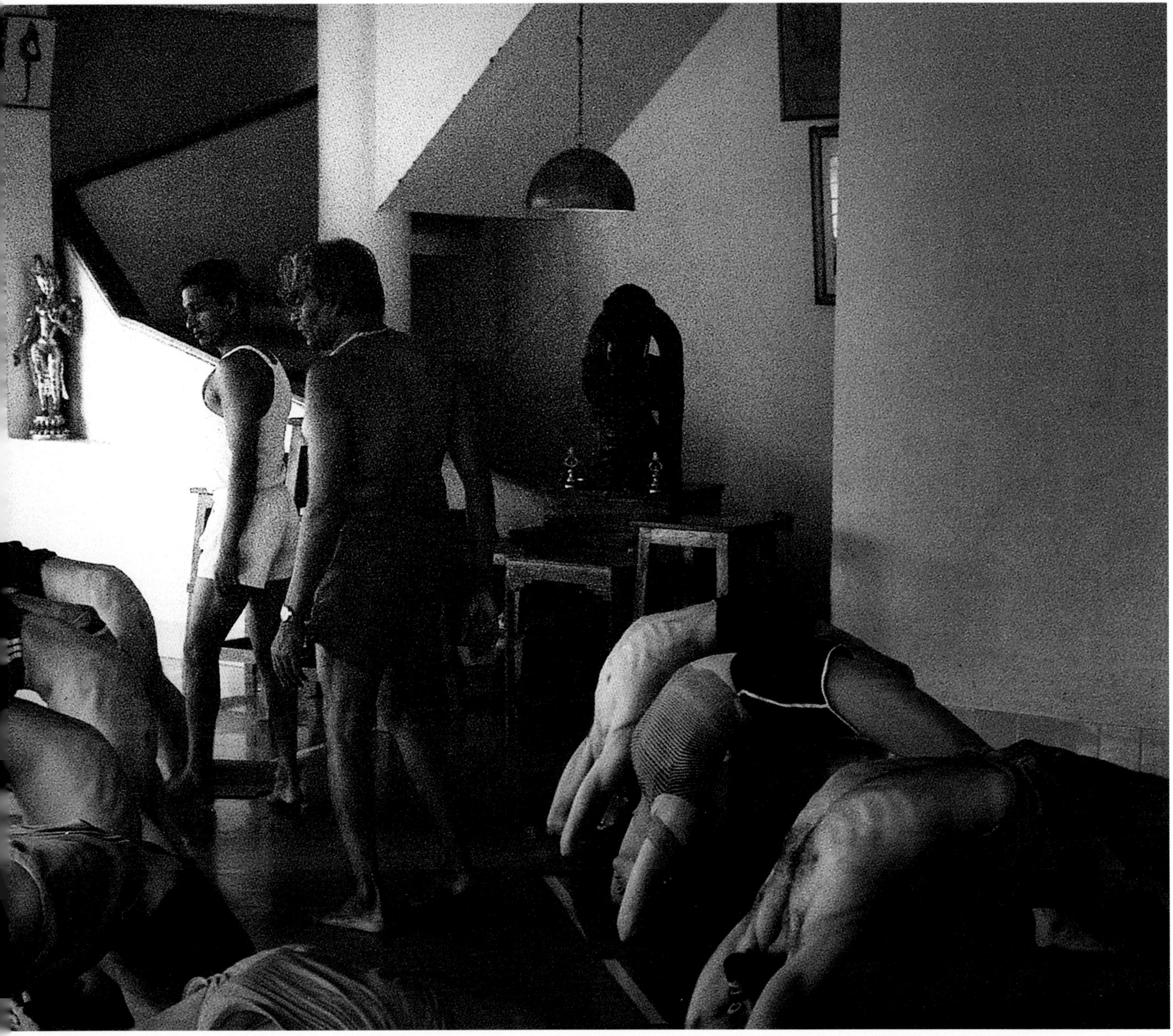

We had Guruji teaching us every morning and afternoon. He would have us do a more general standing pose session, and then every day he would take us through backbends or balancings, or both. One day at the end of a big backbend class he roared, "NOW 50 *VIPARITA CHAKRASANAS*" and left... we actually did them, from the stage, most of us.

We would eat, nap and go back for more. It was the most demanding time I have ever spent, but also the most rewarding mind/body changing time of my life.

PL

Once I was doing *Viparita Chakrasana*, standing and going back and lifting the legs up in handstand and again. We would do 108 every Friday. I had tried for so long, 1½ years. One day I finally got it. I was alone in the yoga hall and suddenly the sound came, "You've got it!" Guruji was on the balcony of the house and he saw me. I didn't know he was there, I was just feeling happy that I got it that day. I thought I'm alone in the hall, nobody saw me, but that's OK. But he saw me from there and he shouted so loudly! I had been very close to getting it before and suddenly that day I got it.

VD (Vinod Dulal)

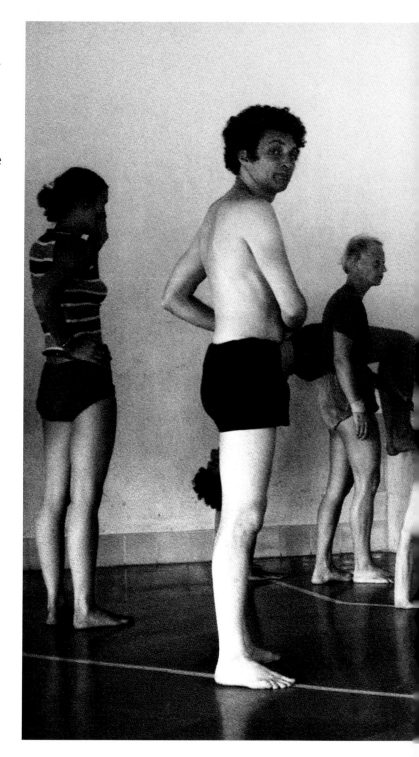

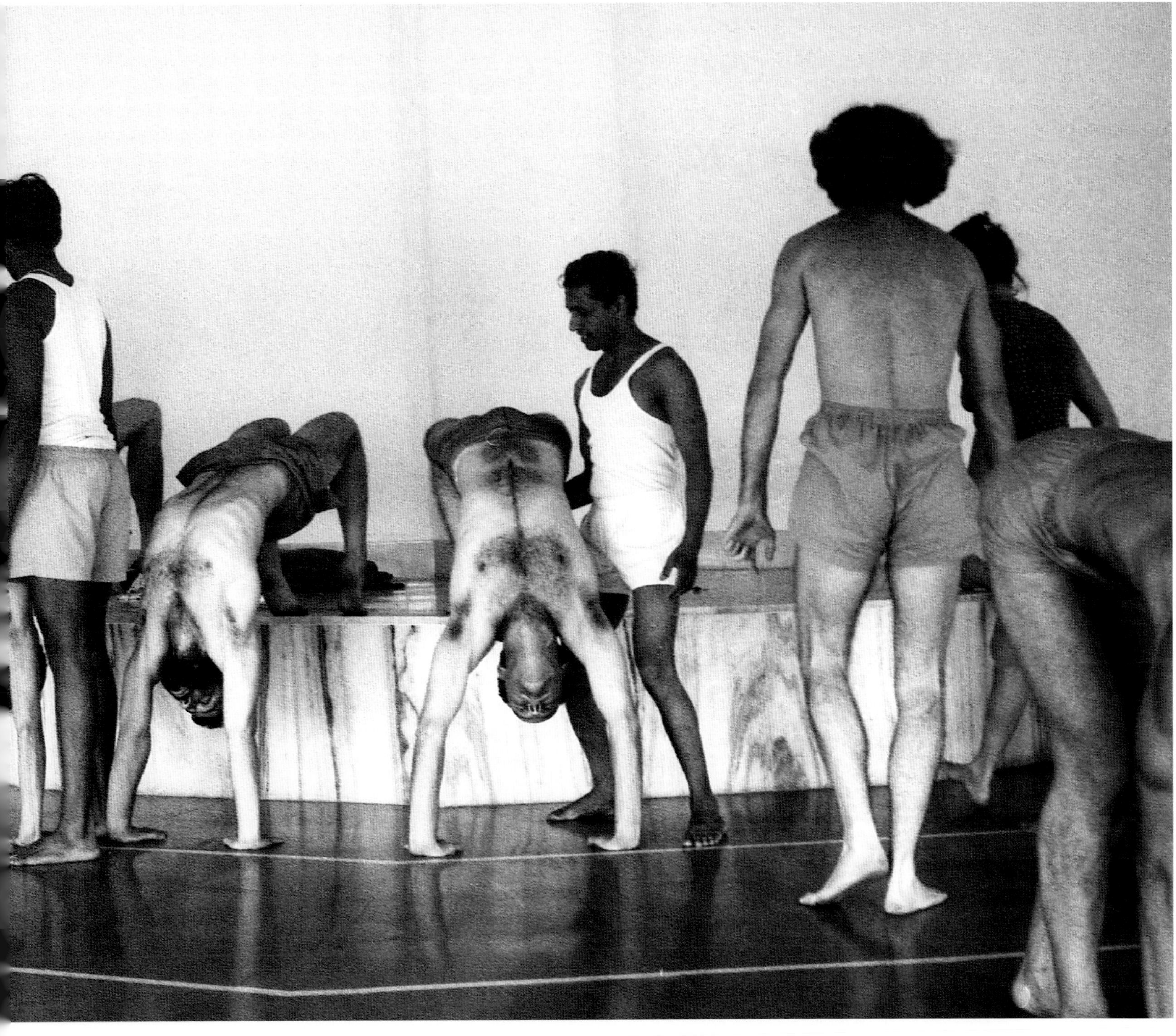

Classes started with almost a week of jumpings, perhaps to tone us and get us moving, get us out of our heads. And then at the end of those first days Guruji suddenly said our eyes were dull and we couldn't learn anymore for that day. He gave us 20 minutes of supported *Halasana* and sent us home.

PL

In the early days, one year we were there between two intensives. That's when I first learned the balancings. Although at the time this was a profound experience, I didn't really understand just how special those tiny classes were.

BC (Bobby Clennell)

Occasionally the weeks were quiet with no major course and perhaps only ten people present at the daily work that continued unabated. Imagine the privilege of working in such a small group with the world's leading exponent of both the practice and teaching of yoga.

AC (Alan Cameron)

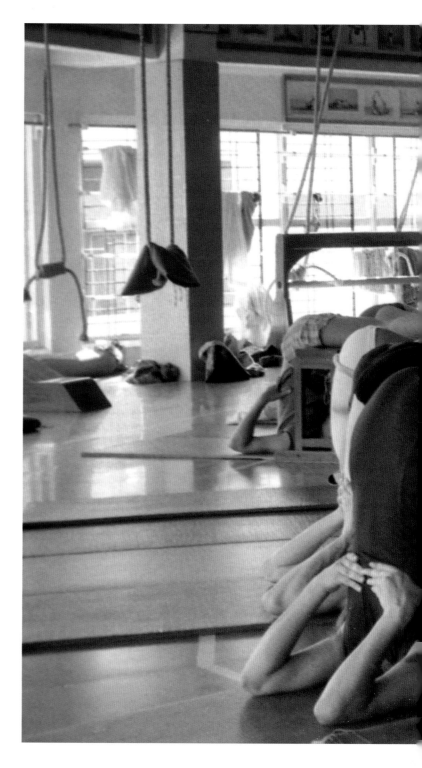

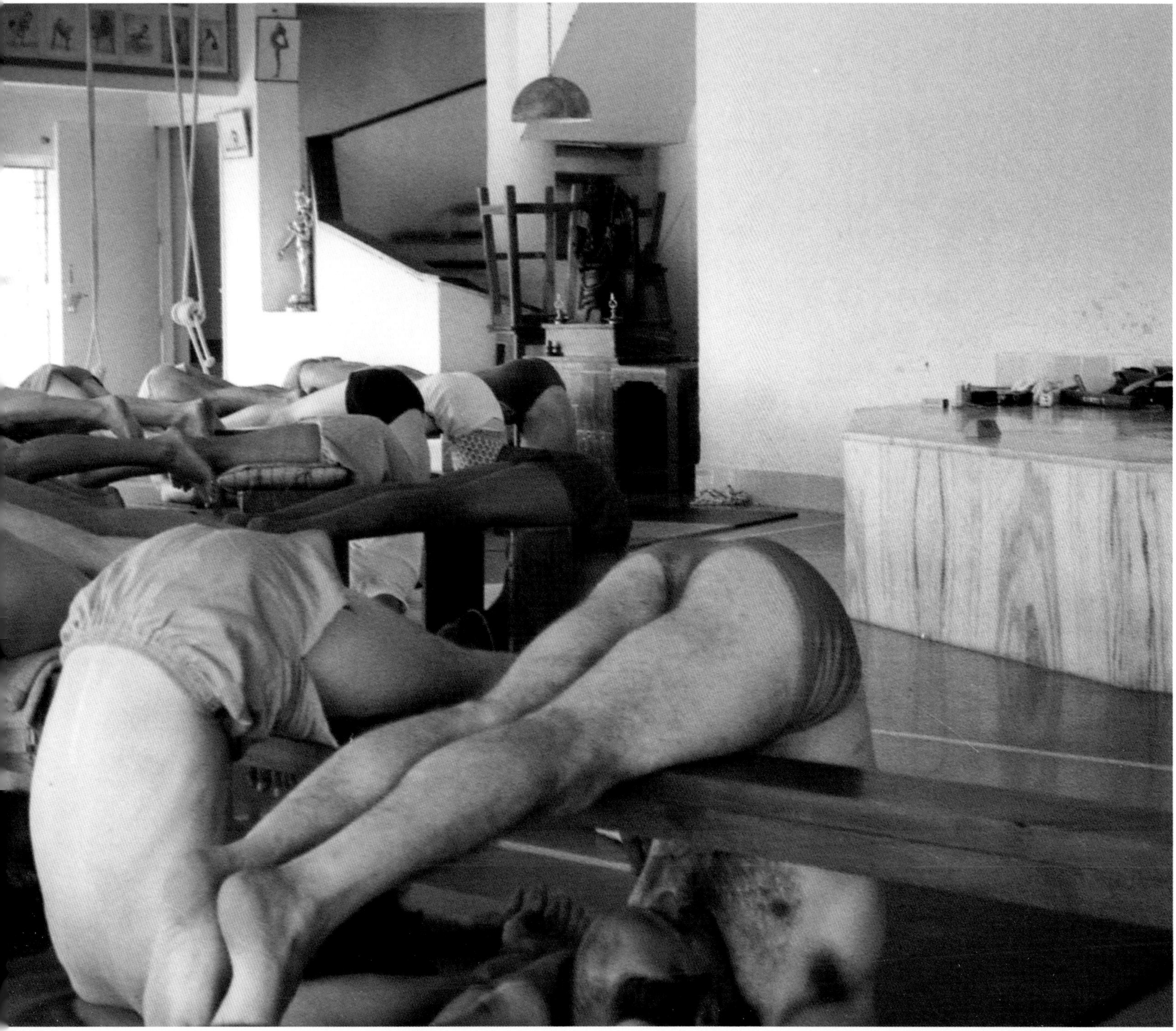

In the early days it was a very different experience. The amount of work he could get out of us was huge. Sometimes he did not give an explanation—all he said was, "Surrender!" and automatically your body surrendered. He could do anything he wanted. The body just gave in. Or he would just put a finger on a muscle here or there and without us knowing it, that muscle would follow his instructions. There was such a lot of communication and understanding between the teacher and the student.

NK (Navas Kamdin)

For all of Guruji's intensity in the class and despite his presence being huge, when he was teaching in some ways he disappeared. He managed to take you right inside yourself and allowed you to experience something deep, in every pose. You got something, perhaps a sense of your own potential. He opened a door that you hadn't even suspected existed, and that captivated us; it captivated me.

It was always about yoga. At the end of the class we would sometimes go up to thank him. I remember him often saying, "Don't thank me, thank yoga." He just wanted you to get a glimpse of the vastness of the subject and where it could lead you.

PL

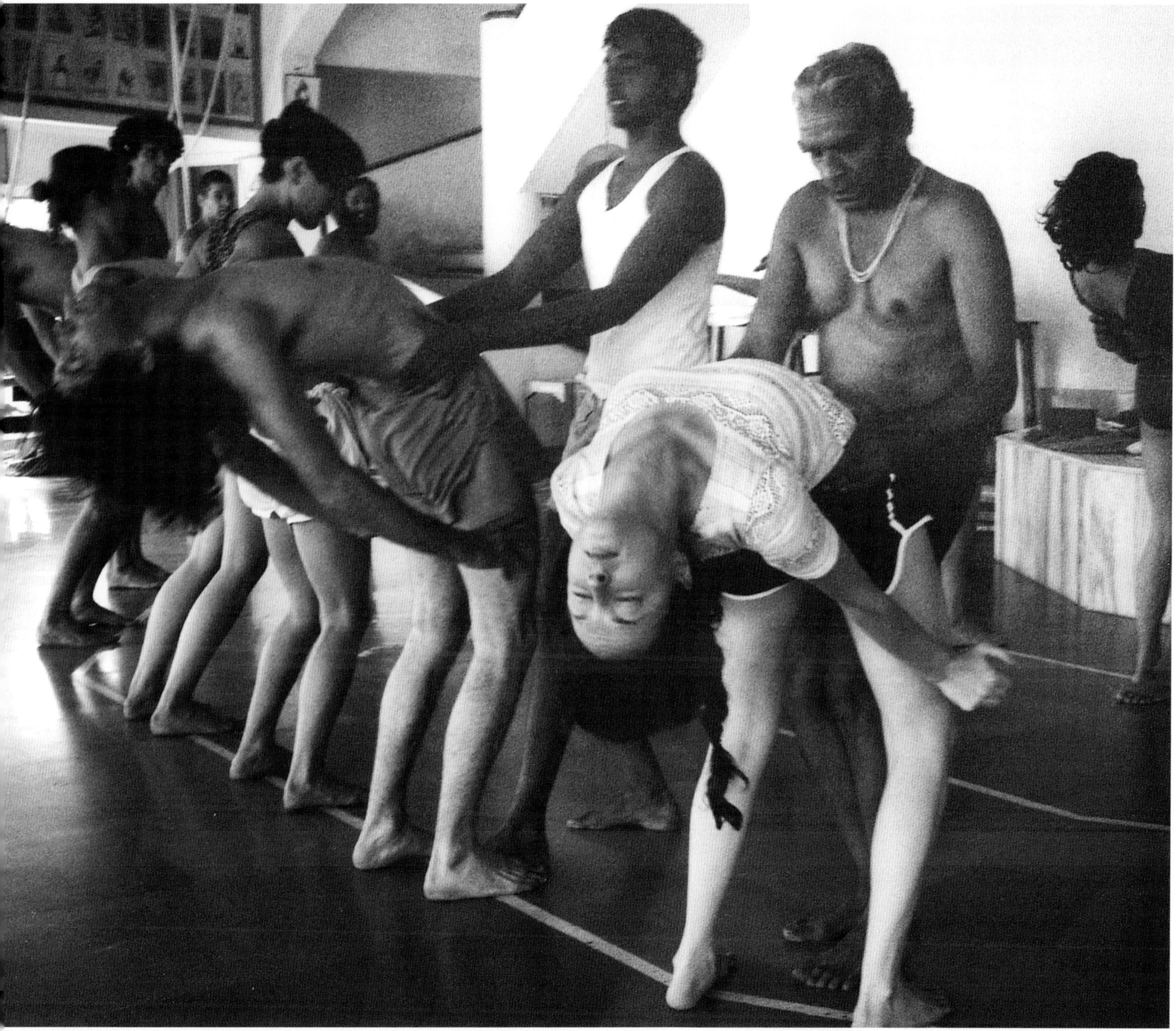

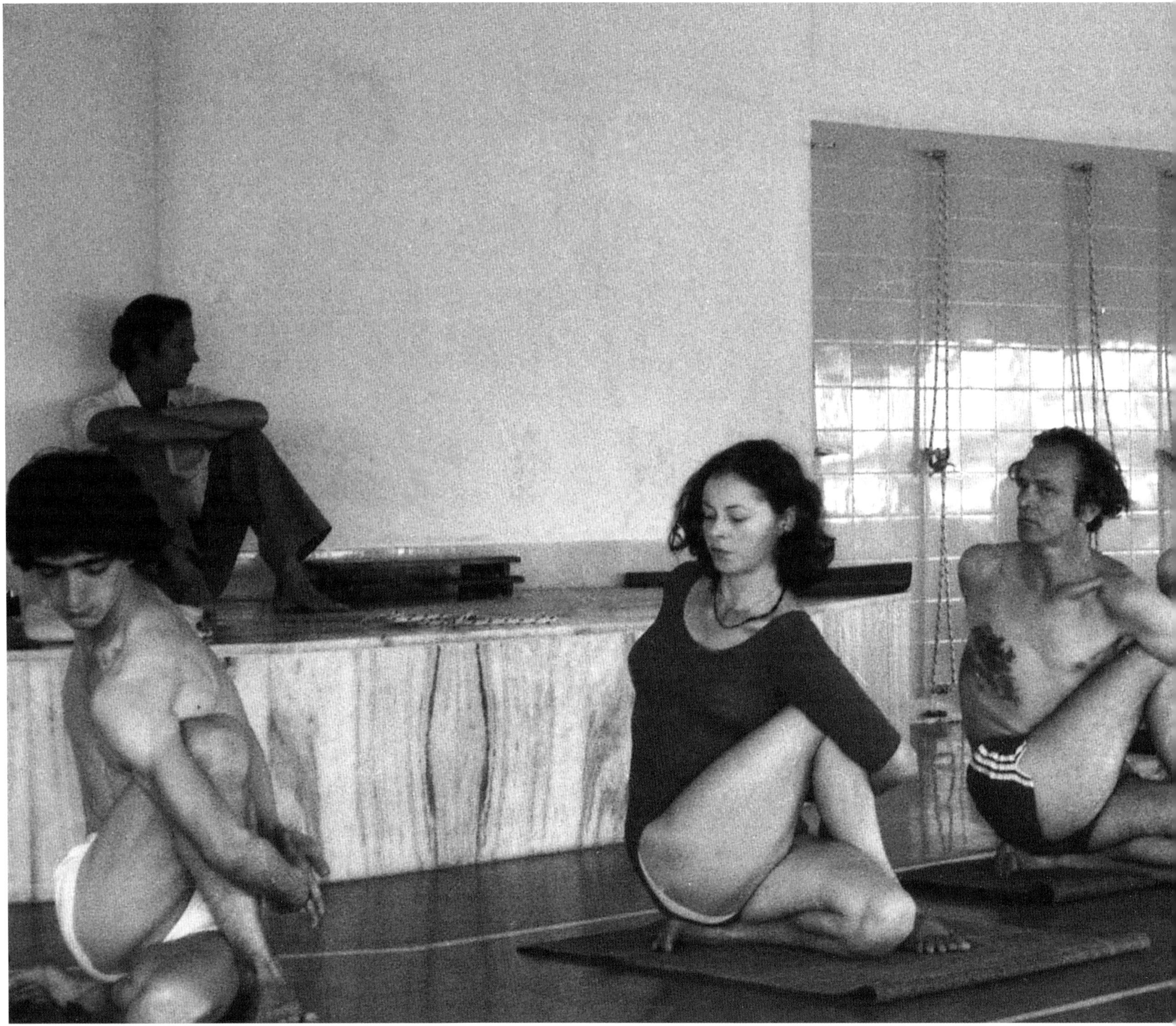

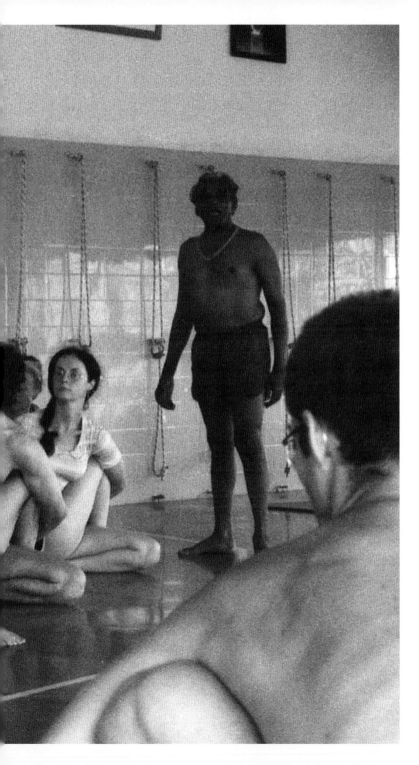

We were just a few students in the class, so whether it was standing poses, forward bends or twistings, he could press each and every one of us. In the twistings—turn and turn and twist and twist—we saw stars! And in *Paschimottanasana* he would be sitting on us and the more we got restless and wanted to get up, the more comfortable he would make himself as if he was sitting on the sofa.

He had a very impish sense of humour. He knew how to make you laugh. He knew how to make you cry. He knew how to relax you.

He had such amazing insight. You only had to come walking up to him and he would tell you what your problems were. What he always told us was, "To be a teacher, be an observer. First observe the way they walk, the way they move. Then only will you understand."

He knew the human body and mind like no one else. And now you have people who try to copy him. It doesn't work at all. He was too good. He was an artist, he was a scientist, he was a teacher, he was a father, a mentor—everything.

NK

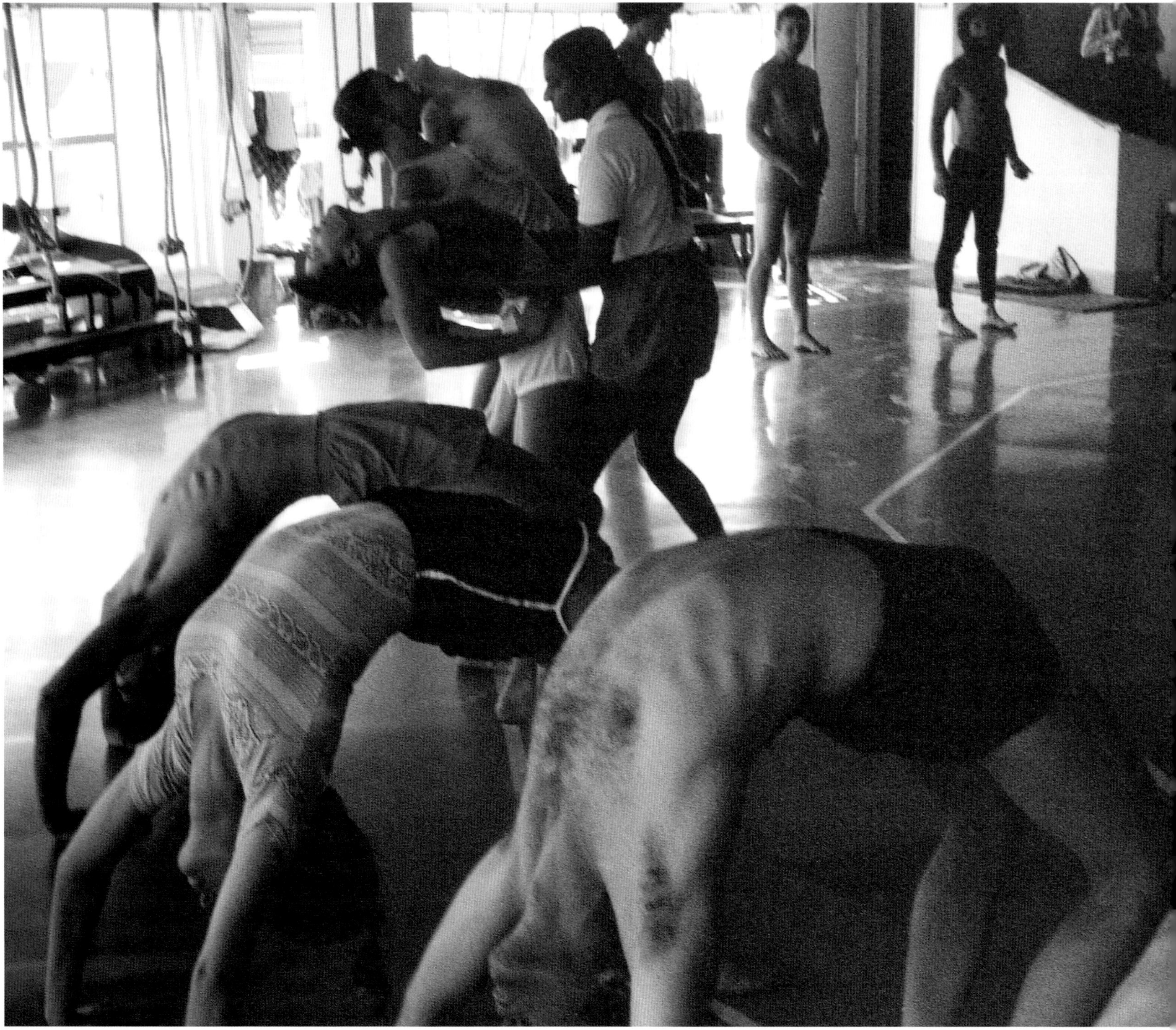

No two classes ever seemed to be the same in any way, except in intensity. The extraordinary atmosphere that was generated at all times literally shaped and enriched people's lives. It is difficult to overstate the privilege of being allowed to practise week after week in that environment.

AC

A significant early memory was my 4th lesson when Guruji asked me to kick up my leg for a full arm balance. I was terrified, but in good faith I kicked up, probably barely lifting 6 inches off the ground. I felt a very quick, sure and strong hand catching my ankle and hoisting me up into the pose and he said to me, "Good." Next he asked a young girl my age, who had joined classes on the same day as myself, to do the same act. She was terrified and refused to attempt. Thereafter, that girl never returned to the classes... I continued...

There could be an element of fear in some students because he would immediately notice lapses, errors and the slightest smack of falsehood, and he was fiercely intolerant of these.

The teaching was brilliant and unparalleled. He had me riveted to yoga for over 40 years. I would be ashamed to show up for my weekly class if I had not practised during the week. But we soon learned that skipping a class was a worse option.

SC (Swati Chanchani)

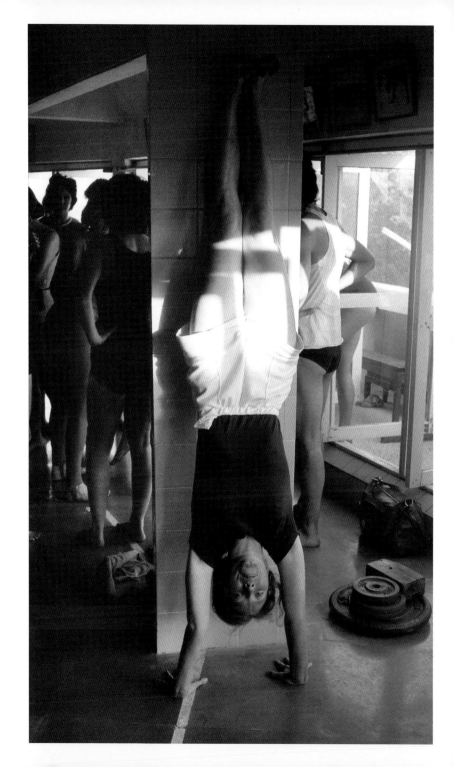

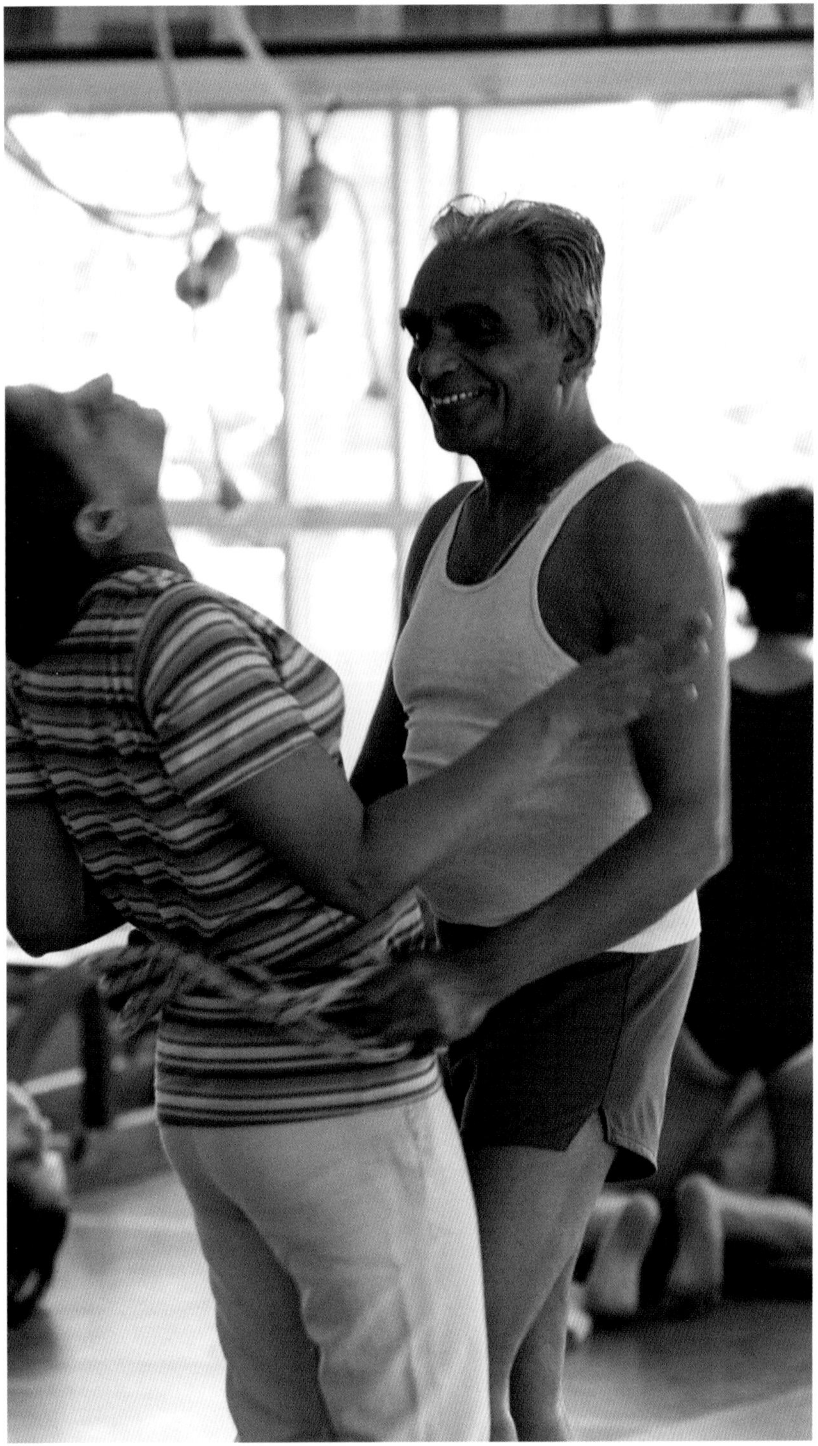
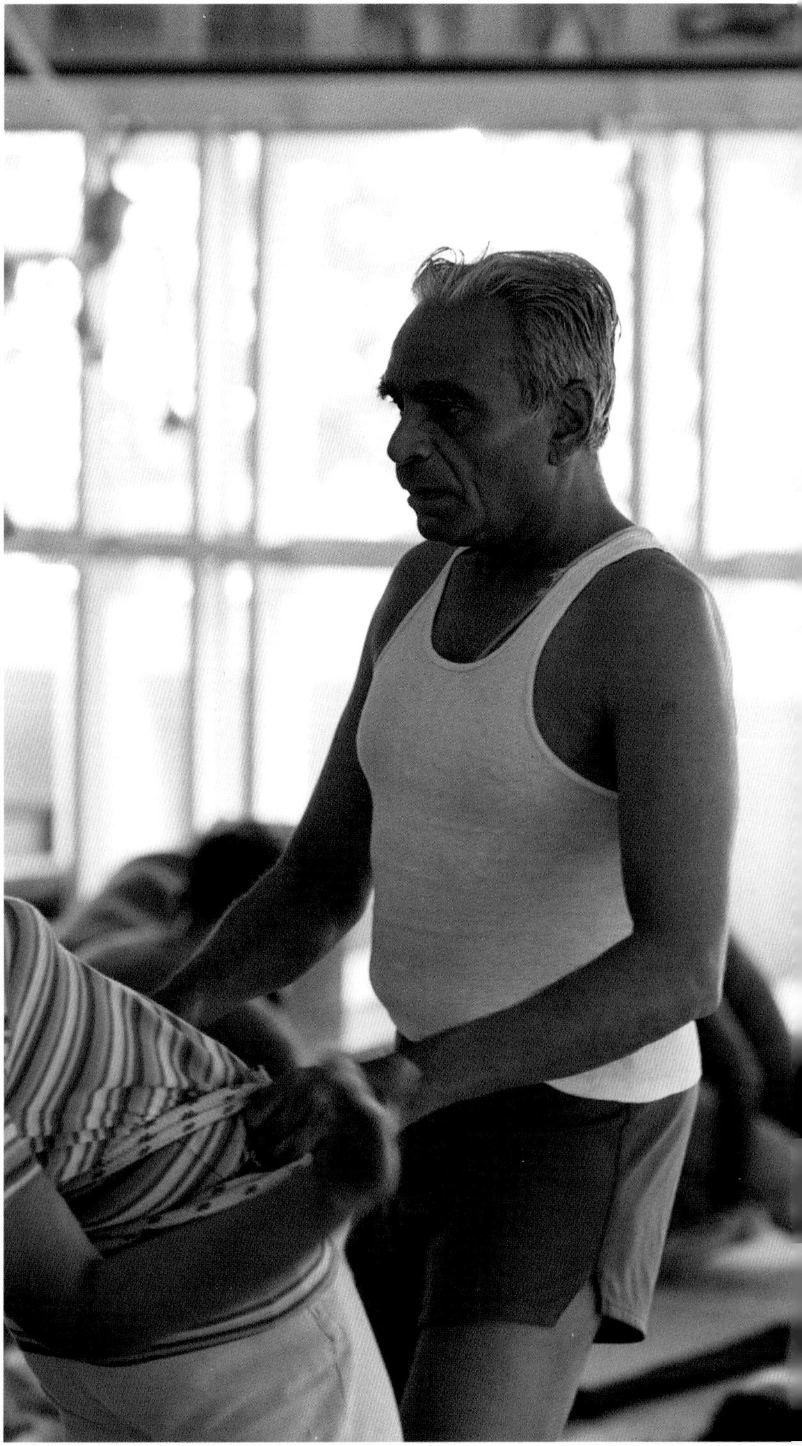

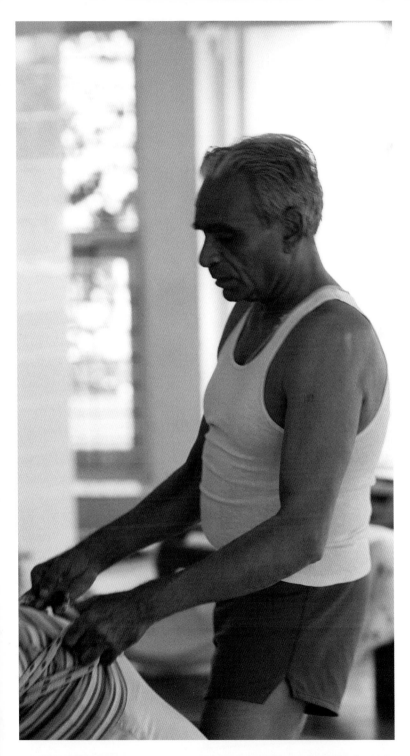

It was so often the case that a great deal of laughter was involved, which was another kind of intensity that Guruji readily engendered.

AC

He showed us early on that he had a sense of humour in those classes, which was endearing and important because it made him approachable. His teaching was so dynamic and he tempered this with his sense of humour. I have a photograph of him from the '70s on which he wrote, "May this laugh inspire you in yoga." He was serious but also lighthearted with his twinkling eyes.

JW

He would say, "To work hard, you must have a sense of humour!"

JP (Julia Pedersen)

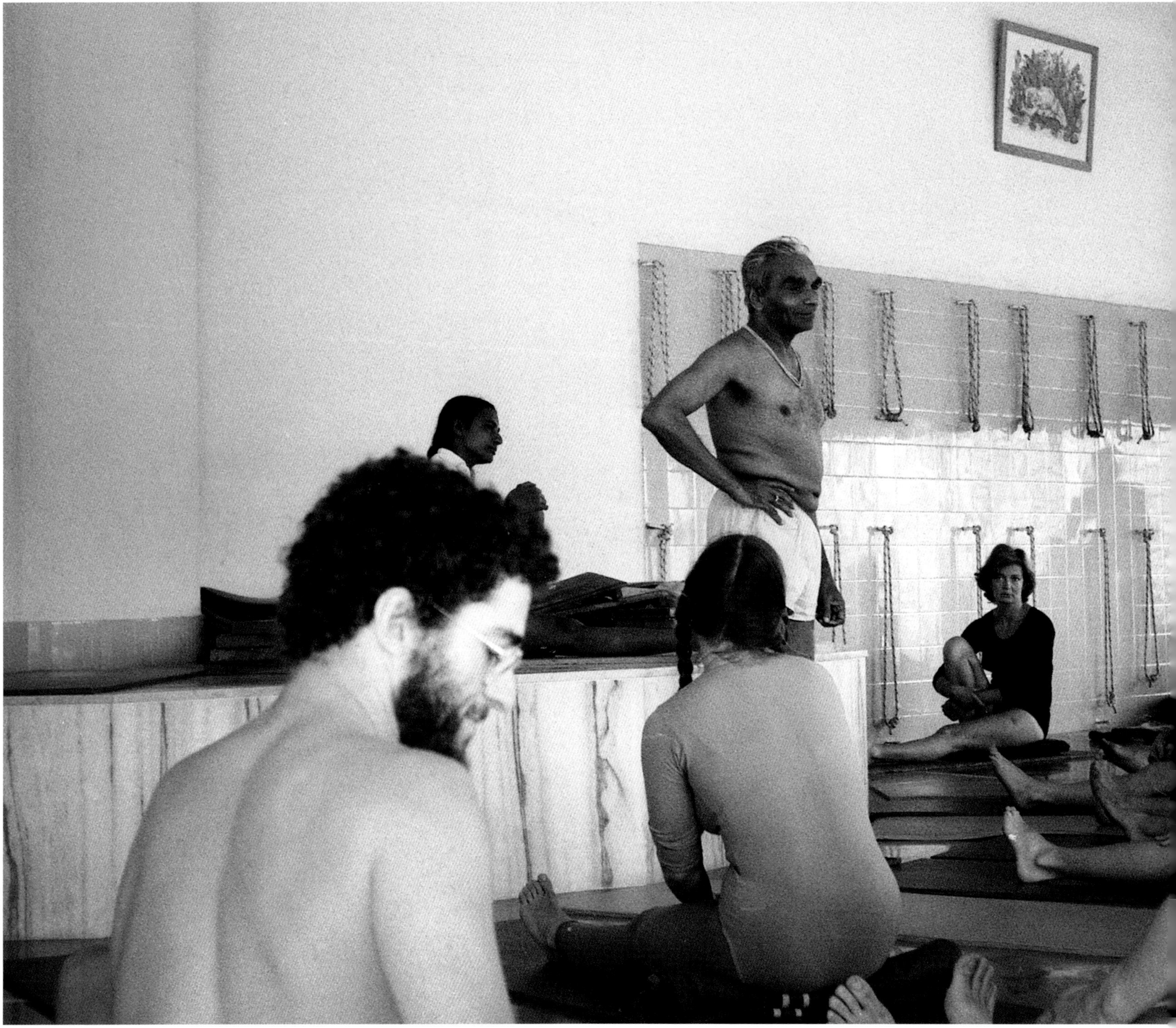

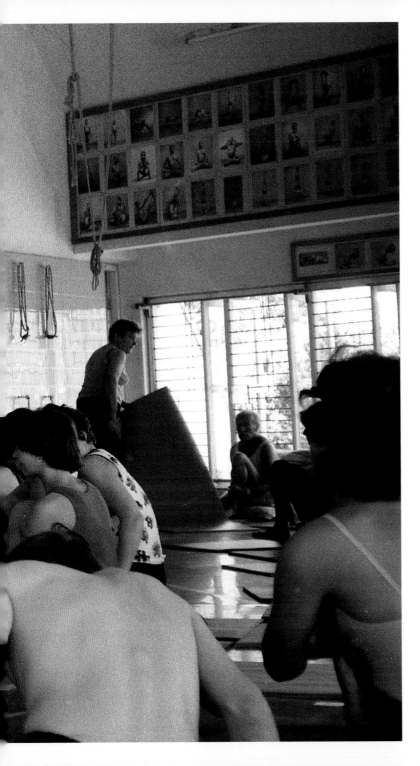

It was crucial to pick up very quickly how to learn—from the basics of respecting the physical environment of the Institute to the subtle complexities of being allowed to observe the amazing weekly remedial class on Wednesday evenings. We Westerners were not in the main a very skilled group, it seems; even such practices as getting out the equipment could all too frequently reveal our inability to co-operate or to listen precisely to instructions. Worse still, on occasion a wooden brick might be dropped on the beautiful polished stone floor—bringing the heartfelt reprimand, "Break your head but don't break my floor!" from Guruji or Geeta. In these and a host of other ways, the daily instruction in *Yama* and *Niyama* would go on in an uninterrupted flow.

Eventually, even the slowest and most clumsy might begin to cotton on to what life in the Institute demanded—and then, to what that life enabled to unfold in any pupil who found a way of really listening. He was meticulous in explaining all aspects of yoga in depth and detail, but equally meticulous in not allowing any form of lazy, self-deluding shortcuts from his pupils.

He maintained a pure, simple and rigorous approach that made the subject accessible to all.

AC

It was electrical going into that first class. He was head and shoulders above what I understood at that moment what humans could be. He pulled the group in, he worked it. He had an extraordinary authority; he had an extraordinary way of understanding of how to work with us. We were held and we were with him entirely. We were held in his hand and we worked at whatever level we were at. I understood I was starting to walk on a pathway. This man was teaching me and I felt like bits and pieces of myself were coming together.

CC (Caroline Coggins)

In his classes, no matter if he was teaching or practising, we had no other choice than to give the best of ourselves. Guruji had an energy that was possible to feel, but impossible to describe. As soon as he left the room the energy level was different. It was as if he had his eyes directly on each one of us the whole time. Practising with him, or talking with him, I felt like I had no secrets—he could even see my thoughts. His practice, his *tapas*, the love for yoga brought him to a different level that affected each of us. With him it was possible to go beyond your boundaries. This was Guruji for me.

GG (Gabriella Giubilaro)

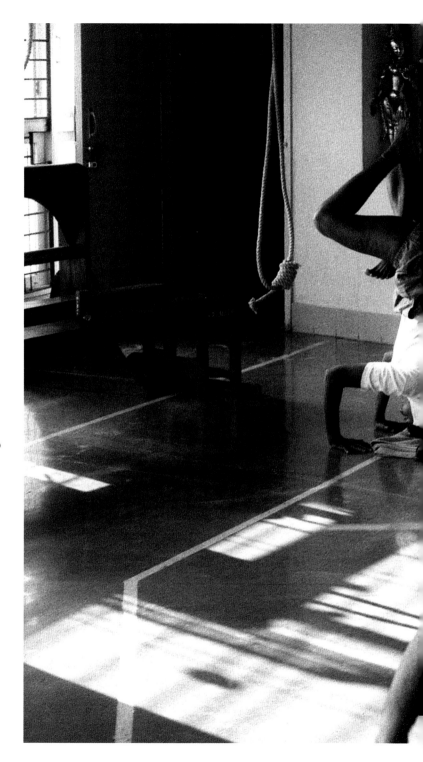

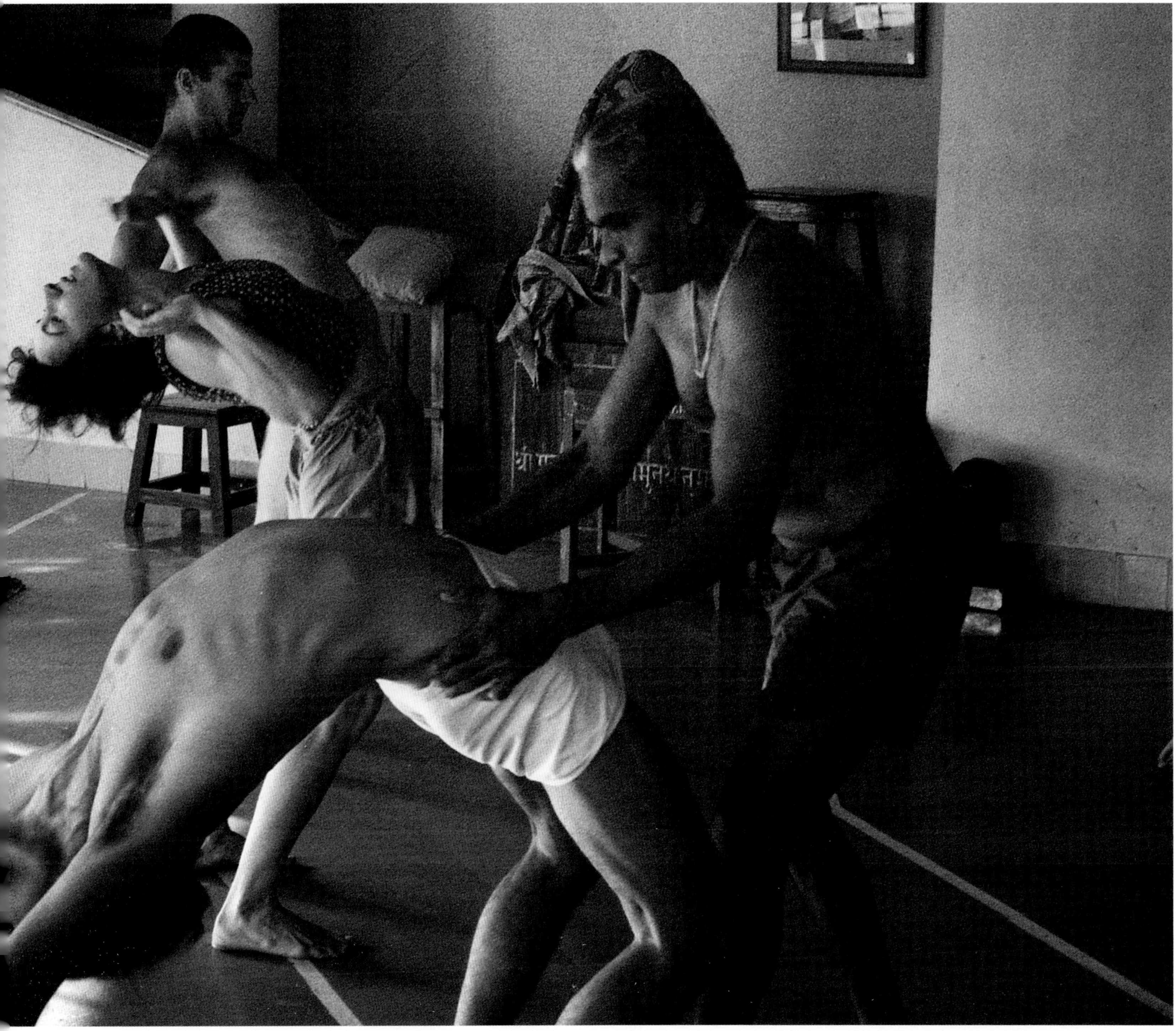

His very personality, his presence, his magnetism were what kept me going. And the creativity! It almost hypnotised me into wanting to go back again and again to see next time, now what?

FAR

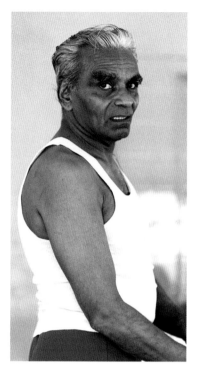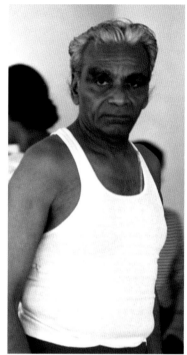

From early on the love was of his art. Yoga was his beloved. He was devoted to his practice, to Patañjali and to his students. He was totally devoted to his students. That was why he was relentless. He really cared. That's why way back we were totally captivated by him. We had never had that experience in a teaching before. He was showing caring by being unrelenting. He wanted to make sure we were understanding.

PW (Patricia Walden)

Guruji was not a mysterious Yogi sitting in a remote cave. He was accessible to us. We saw his ups and downs and watched him face every challenge with equanimity. He showed us how to walk in the world and yet not be of it.

AD

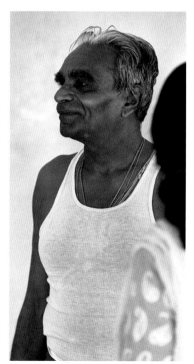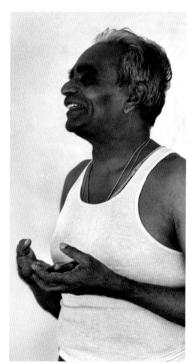

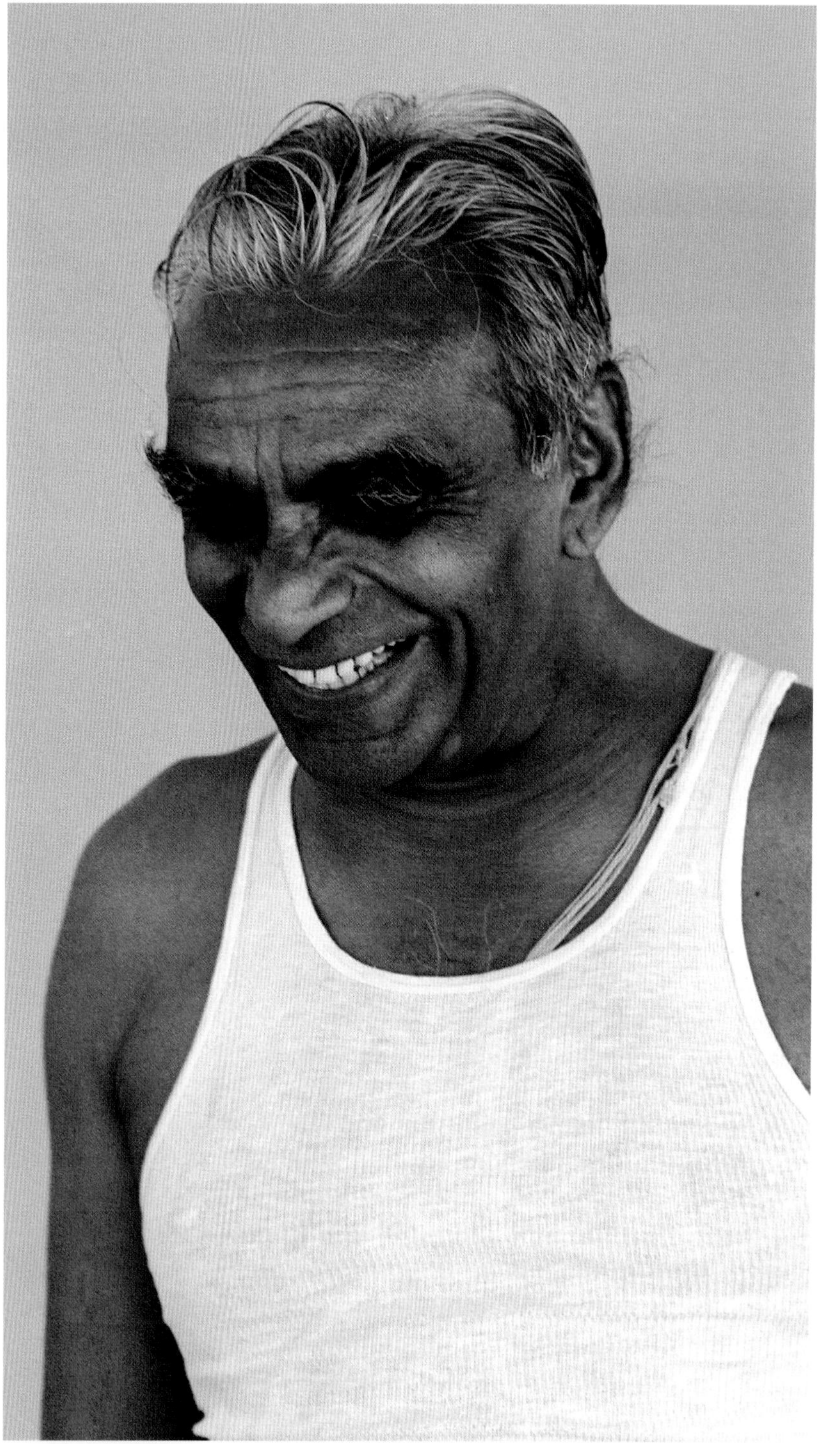
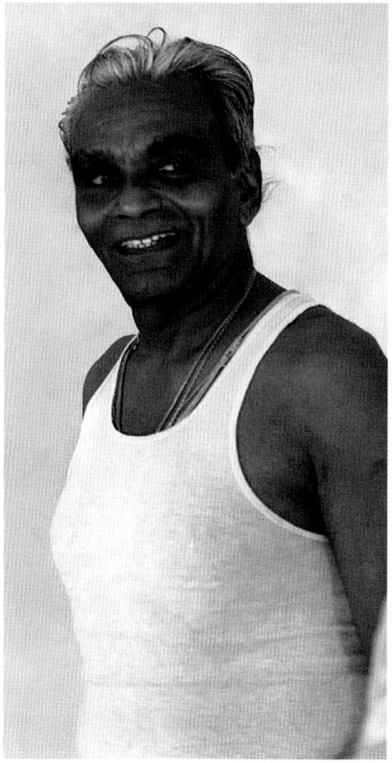
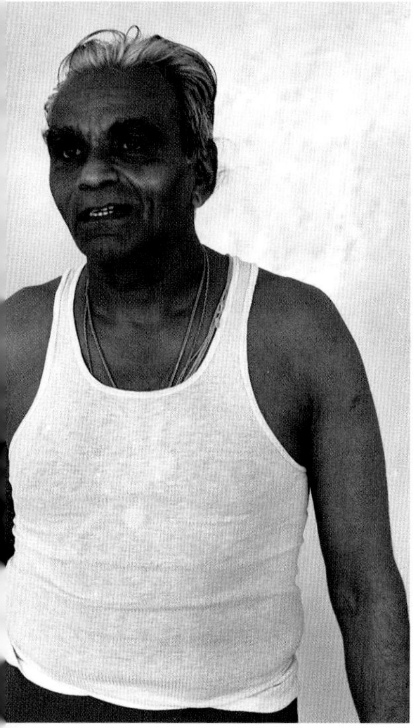
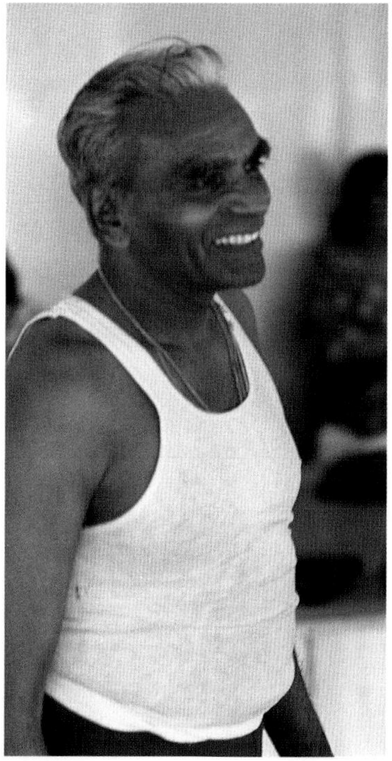
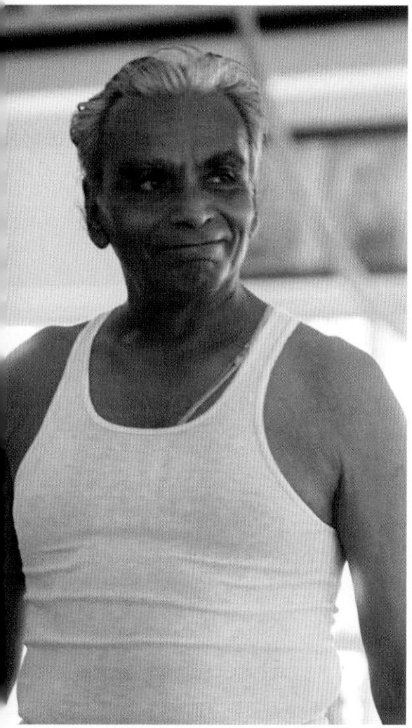

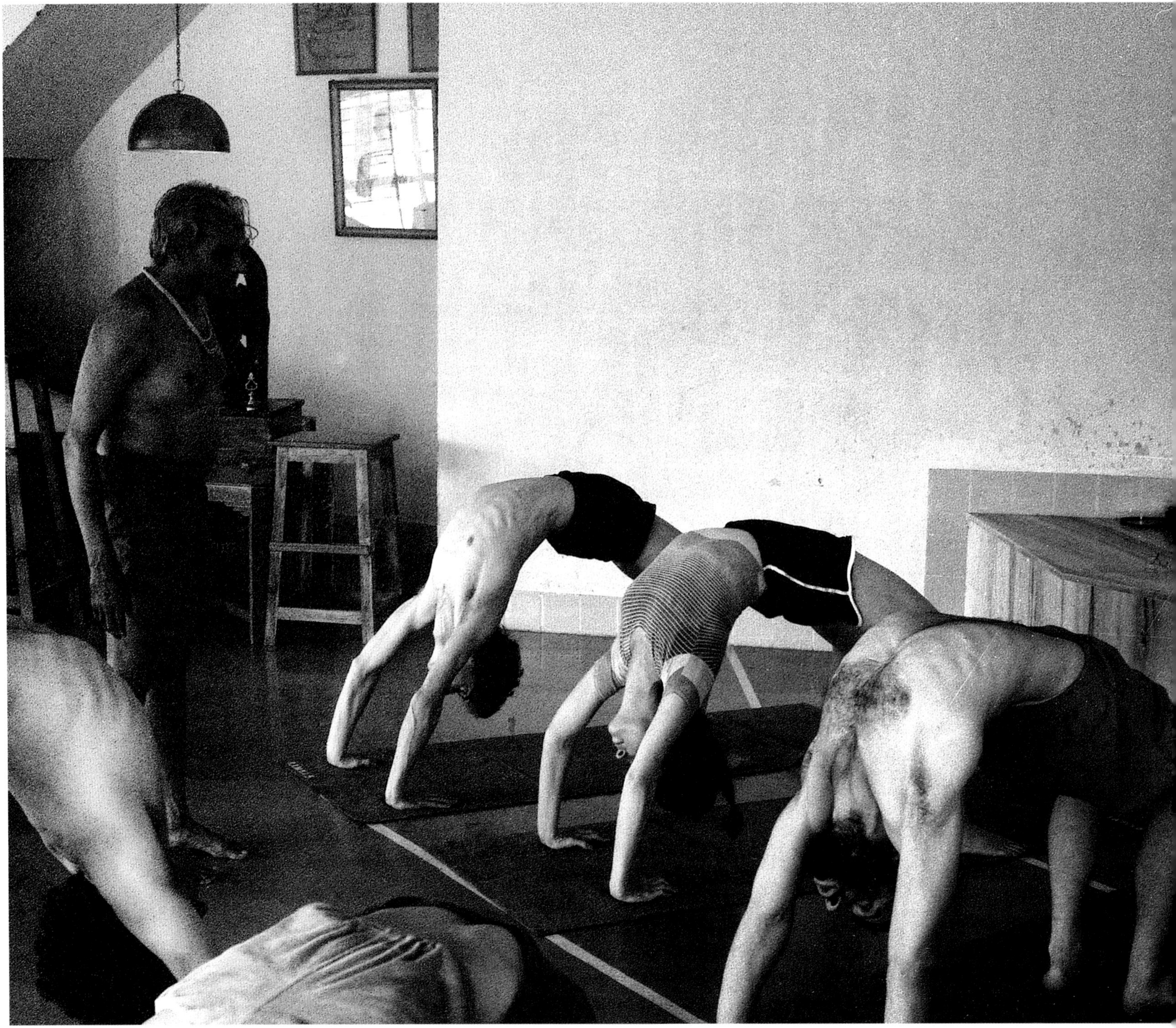

Guruji had a phenomenal ability to 'see' people. There was no escape. All were subject to his penetrating attention. In return he demanded your undivided attention. His teaching bypassed gender, age and class and he made you do things you never imagined you were capable of.

BC

Nothing could have prepared me for that first contact with the Master. Before I had gathered my senses Guruji was standing on my mat, hands on his hips, with his bushy eyebrows and penetrating eyes staring into mine. In full voice he asked, "Who is your teacher?" I could only answer truthfully and said his name. Guruji replied, "Well he knows nothing!" He turned away and continued teaching the class and I was shocked. However, on reflection, I understood his reply was not meant to denigrate my earlier teacher, but instead to make me surrender to Guruji's presence and teaching. Guruji's eyes were everywhere, his voice penetrating and directed at every cell in my body. From that moment I knew I was in the presence of a great man.

KW (Karen Wilde)

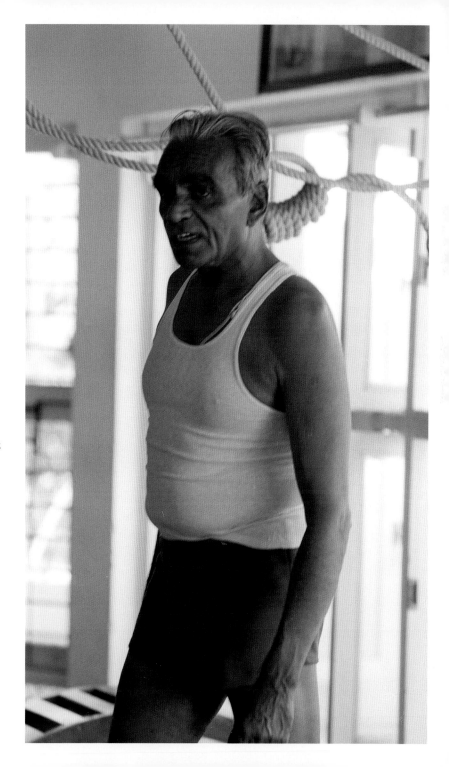

These photos immediately bring to mind what it meant to get Guruji's touch on your body. Whether he came and stood on you, sat on you, adjusted you with a hand or his foot, it would always leave a really deep impression. It helped you to go on. You knew what to do. I remember a time when I was in *Savasana*, it was a *Pranayama* class and he came and adjusted my head with his feet. He lifted my head off the floor and got it just right and I still remember that sensation.

Each and every person he would adjust himself. Only he could make you do all these things. He knew exactly where you should twist and where you should stretch and where you should let go. It was always so special that he would demonstrate everything that he was trying to make you do. I think that is really the mark of a great teacher. They can show you because they practise so much. You can trust them because they know exactly what they are talking about.

AD

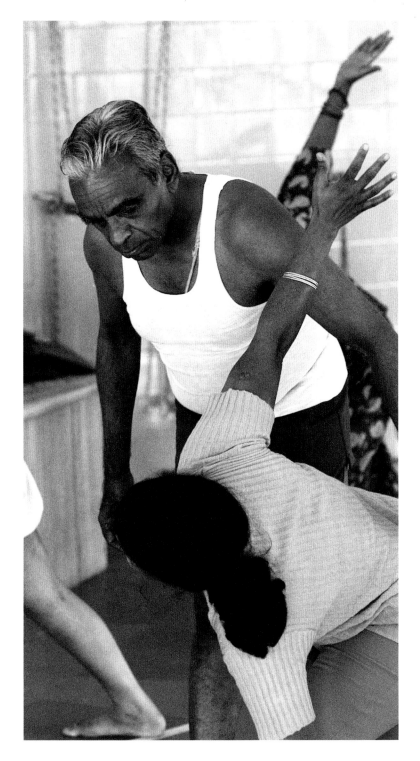

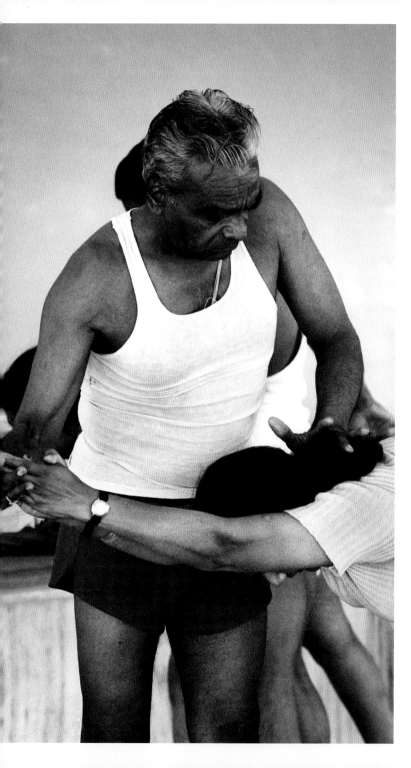

And what did also fascinate me was his touch. His little adjustment. You know, that small turning of your skin— "Stretch here, turn it like that," and that made a whole lot of difference to your balance, to your alignment.

FAR

I remember very clearly that the timings in these supported backbends were often very long with Guruji. You did NOT come up out of the pose before he said to come up. And that realisation made your mind quiet. You gave up your internal struggle and surrendered.

JP

Mr. Iyengar's generosity amazed me. What understanding lay behind his fierceness and intensity as a teacher! It was some years before I came to fully appreciate and to grasp the integration and systematic approach of his teaching. This understanding and intelligent action was utterly transformative for me and has sustained and directed my practice and teaching for over 30 years.

PT (Peter Thomson)

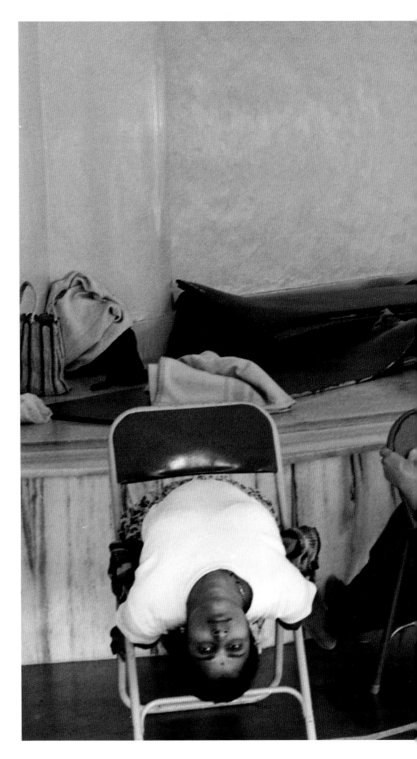

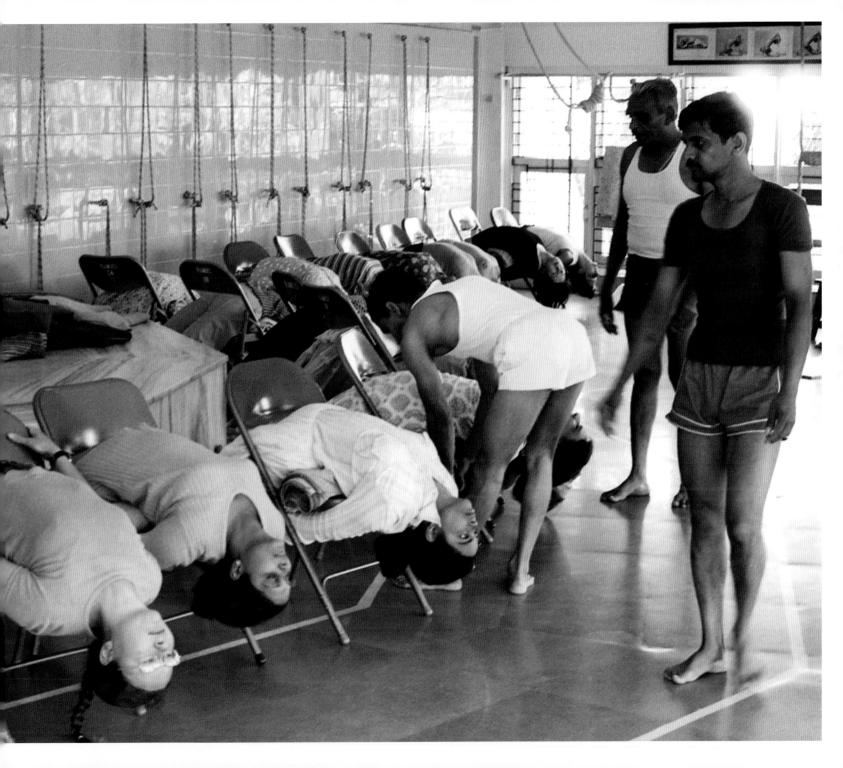

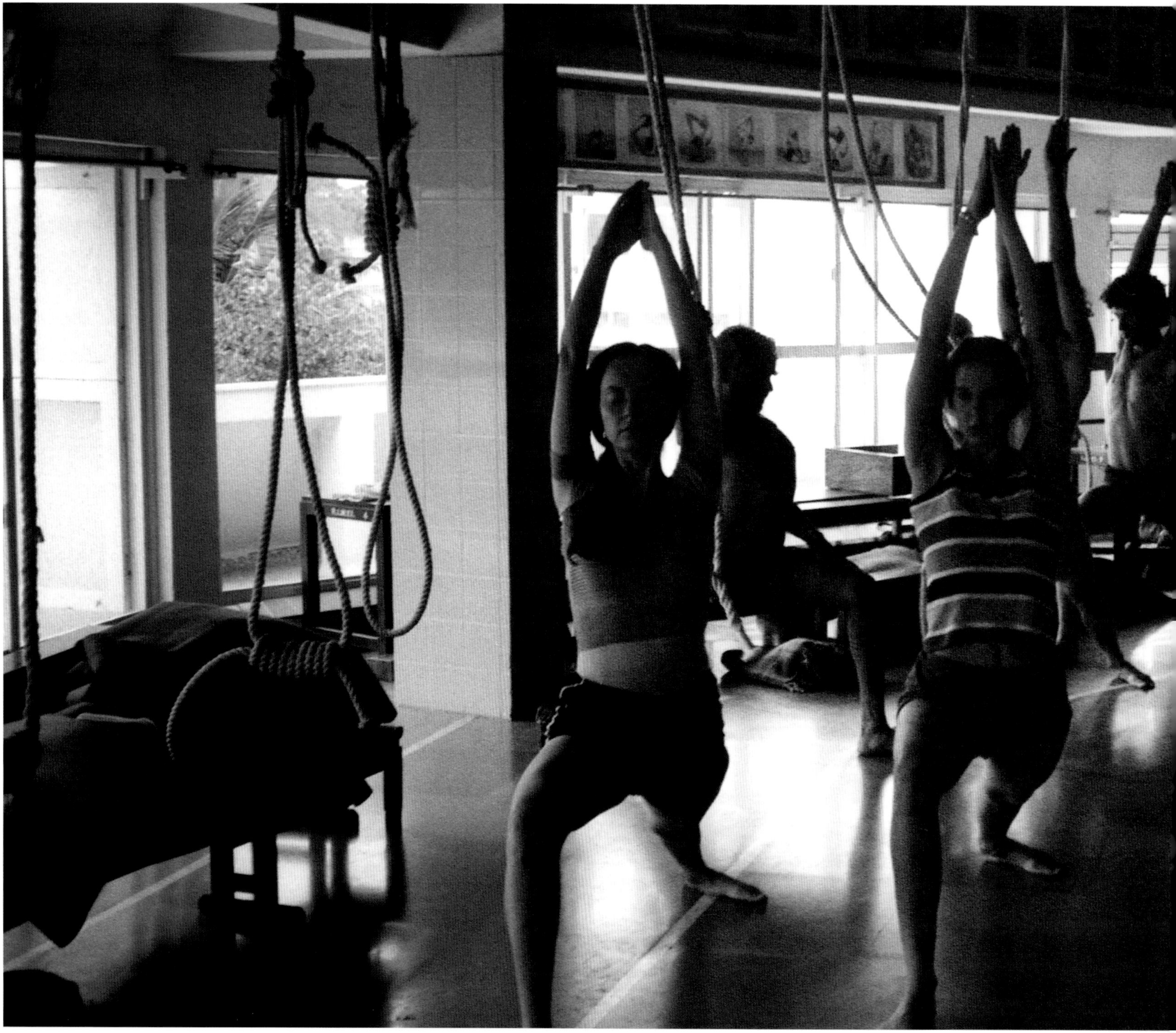

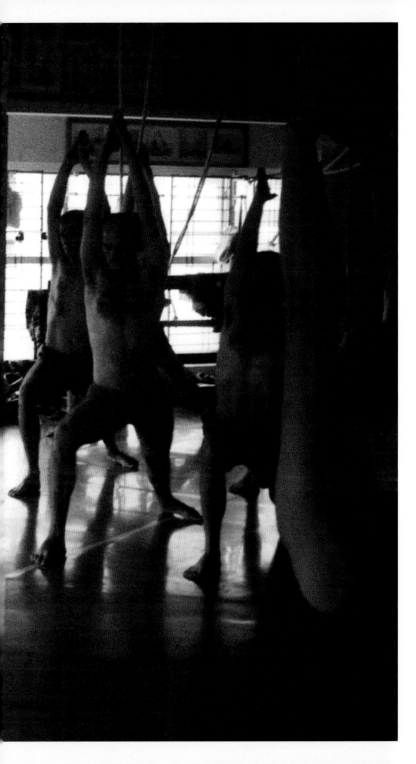

Guruji was teaching standing poses. He was demonstrating *Virabhadrasana II* and he called us all around. He took his hand on his bent thigh and moved it from the knee to the groin. "Did you see what happened?" And we all said, "Yes," so he said, "What was it?" Nobody said anything—because we actually couldn't see it. He did it again. "Did you see?" No one said anything. He wanted us to see how the skin moved. He would get very upset that we couldn't see what he wanted us to see. He would demonstrate something and we didn't have the maturity or skill to see what he was teaching. We couldn't catch as quickly as he wanted us to catch.

PW

I am amazed that we people were being taught by Guruji himself. Nowadays I feel rather sorry that Guruji had to teach the likes of us and not greater talents or more evolved beings.

RAW (Richard Agar Ward)

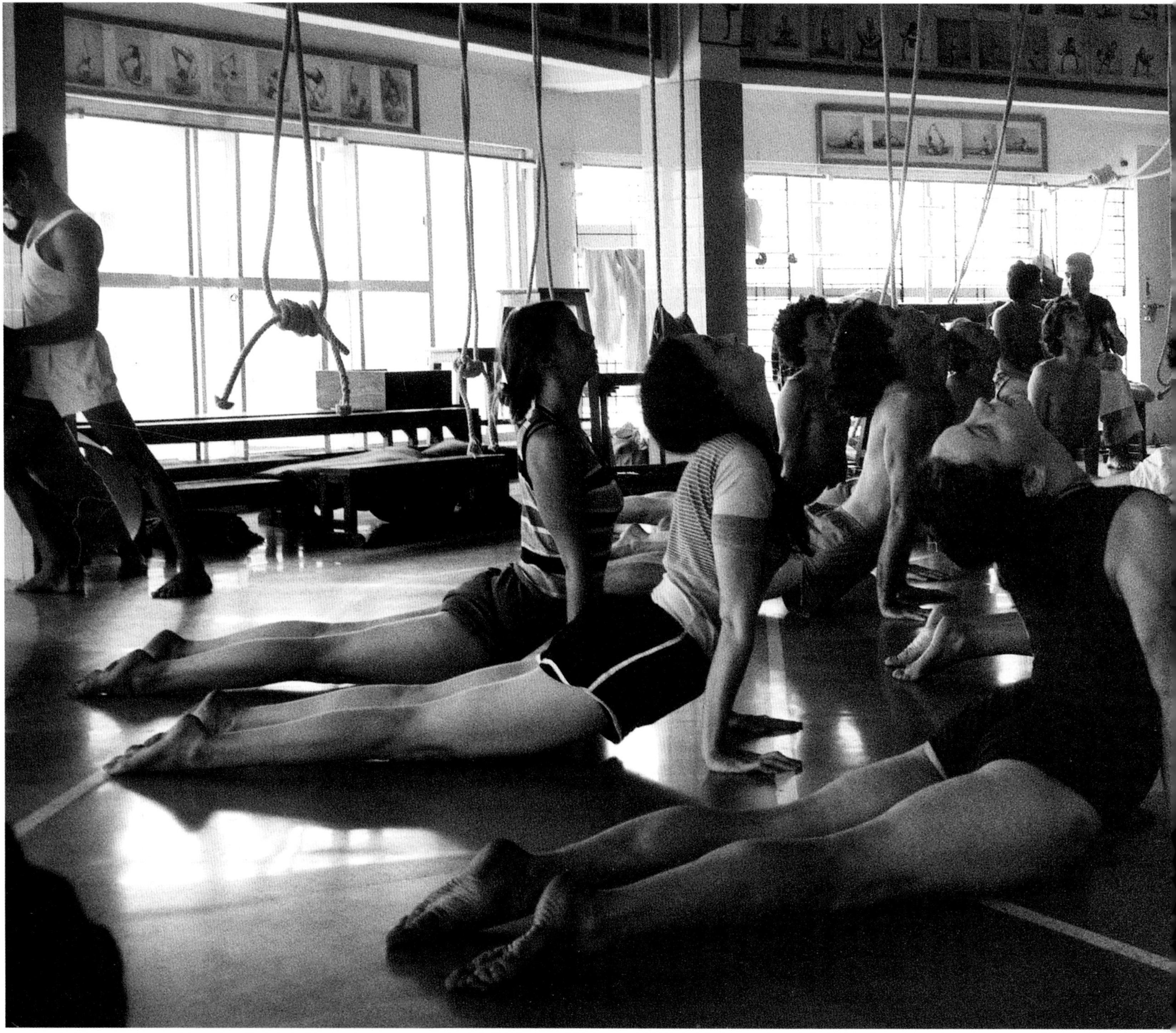

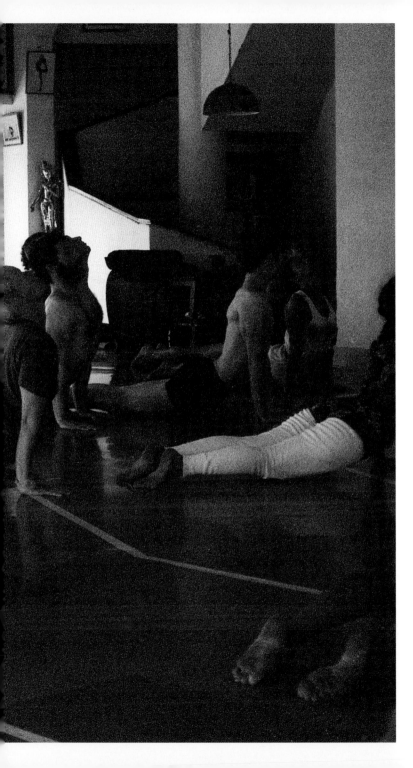

The effect of those early classes on the body was definitely very intense. Something was happening in your brain which you were unaware of.

BM (Birjoo Mehta)

Guruji's classes were very penetrating. They used to reach somewhere deep inside. He made the subject very fascinating. It was never boring and there was no stagnation. There was an ever freshness of the subject. I understand this now. At that time I was not mature to understand all those things. Gradually I started to understand the actions, the penetration, how you have to remain in the reaction.

RN (Rajlaxmi Nidmarti)

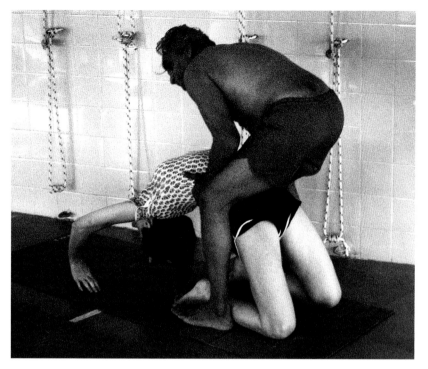

He took 40 people back, some for the first time, into full *Kapotasana*. With lightning speed, he moved along the line and took each student into the complete, final pose. There were surprised and startled grunts as each student just found themselves with their head on their feet. He then walked away and said, "I have given you the pose." He added that now that we had been in it, we had experienced something inside. "Now you have the imprint of the pose, even if it takes you ten years to get back to it." This was the way he worked. He gave you what you needed and then you had to go away and find out for yourself, really learn it. He gave constantly to each and every student, wanting nothing more than for us to 'get it', to glimpse something of what he had experienced with yoga.

PL

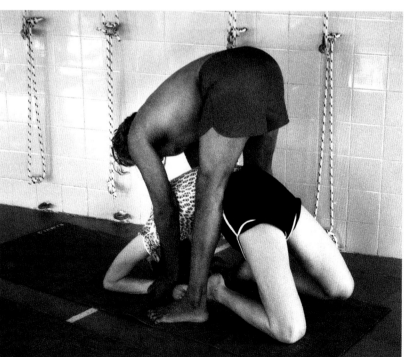

He used to manipulate your body so he didn't need to use words. The effect on the body was definitely very intense. Virtually he used to work with his hands and legs as props. He even used his head.

BM

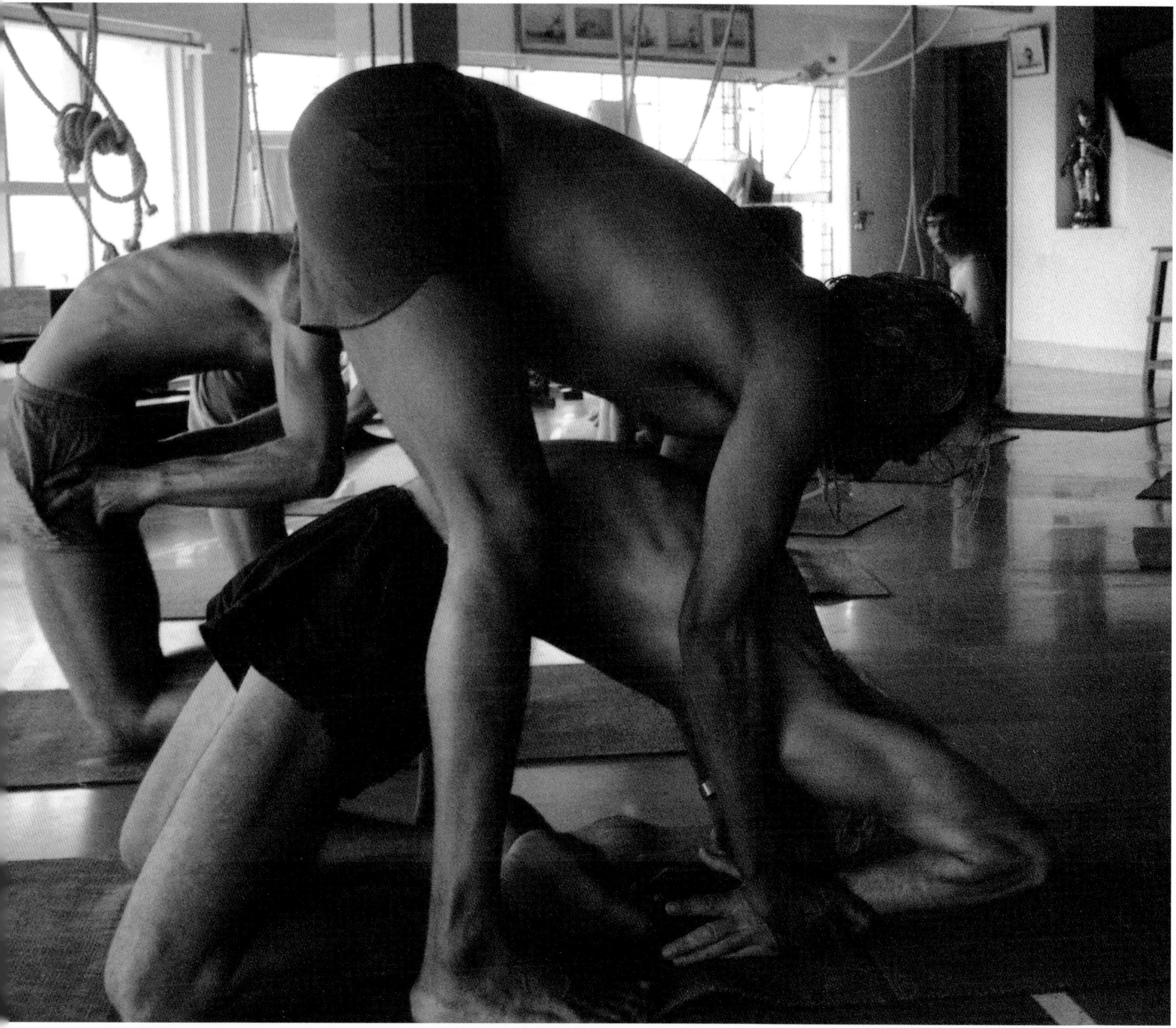

During the monsoon we could be wading through knee deep water at 7 a.m. in the morning to reach his class. I mean, nothing in the world could deter me from going to that class. My family was totally aghast, because I was a person who liked to sleep in late, sleep till half past 7 a.m. What is this thing that is keeping her going and this crazy passion for it?

I'm very glad to have had Guruji as my teacher because we could never ever have our egos up there. Every time something came up it was squashed very instantly. That's very nice because that helped us to understand the essence of yoga, to have to go back for more learning. There is this big danger of thinking that I have arrived or I have become something or I have achieved something. But going back to Guruji each time, going back to Pune and with Geetaji, Prashantji—it's a very humbling experience. I must have displayed my ego at some time, but I know for a fact it would make me re-think and get into myself for more exploration. And that is how I think the journey of yoga has sustained me for so many years. Because yoga is a journey. It never ends.

FAR

Like when you are doing *Setubandha Sarvangasana* for example or *Viparita Dandasana* what he would do is that you would be there and he would lift our legs up, bring his knee below our tailbone and then like a nut-cracker, just push our knees down so that our tailbone is kept on his knees and lifted up and the legs are brought down with that action, giving us that lift in *Setubandha Sarvangasana*. So before the Institute we had absolutely no props at that time, nothing.

In *Sarvangasana* for example if he had to adjust, we didn't really have that many blankets, we had about 2 blankets each—if he had to adjust, he would lift us up and put our shoulders on his feet, lift us up in *Sarvangasana* so that our shoulders are up from the blankets, insert his feet underneath, both feet and then he would slowly bring us down so that we are on his feet and then he would pull his feet back so that the skin on the shoulders also moves back and then we are right on top of the shoulders, the front end of the shoulders and not on the back end of the shoulders. Those kinds of adjustments he would do.

BM

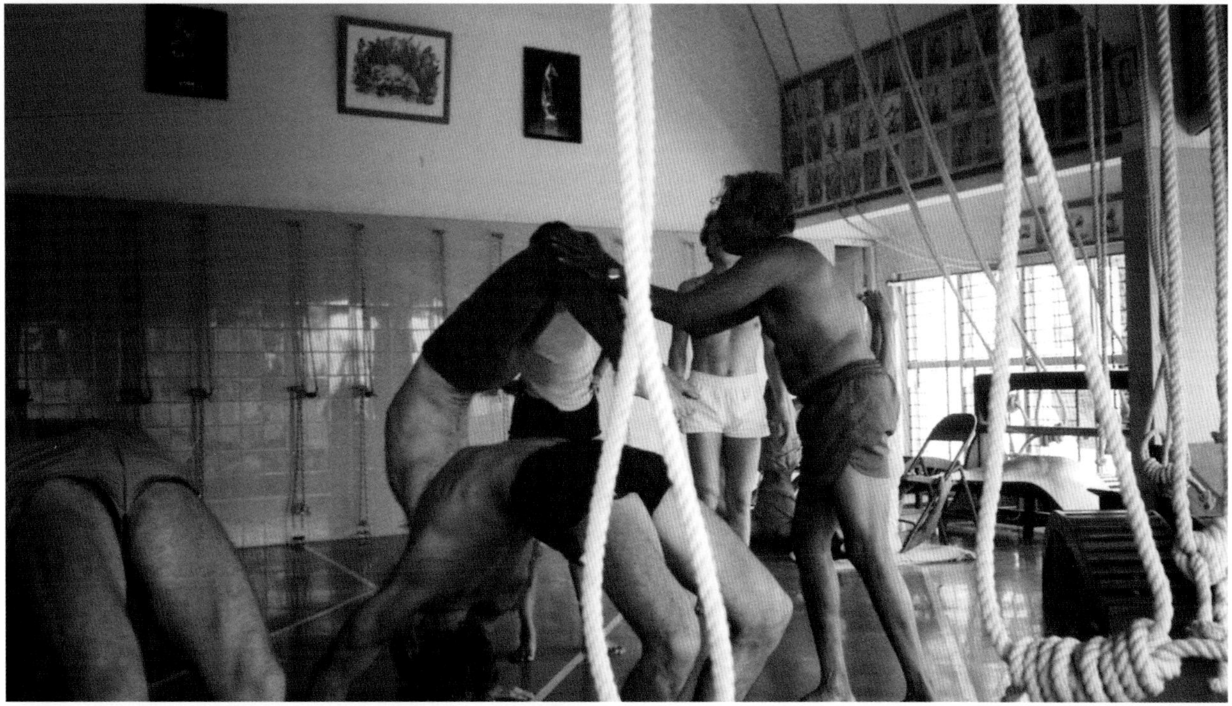

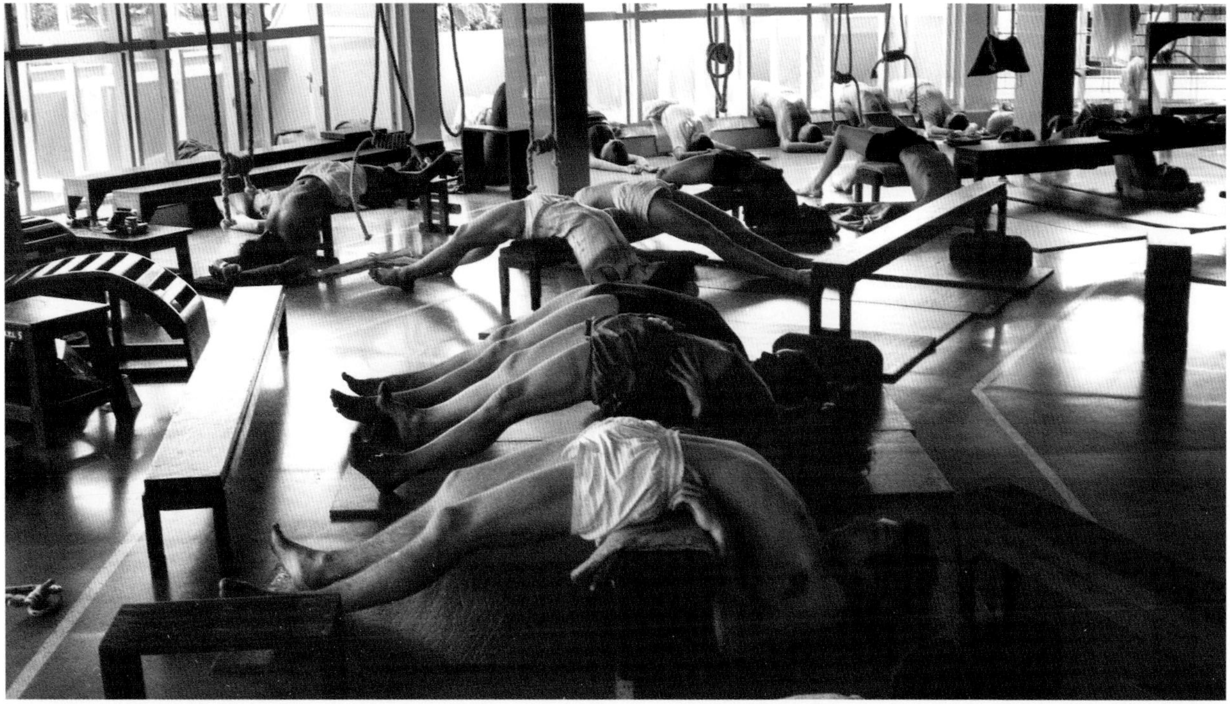

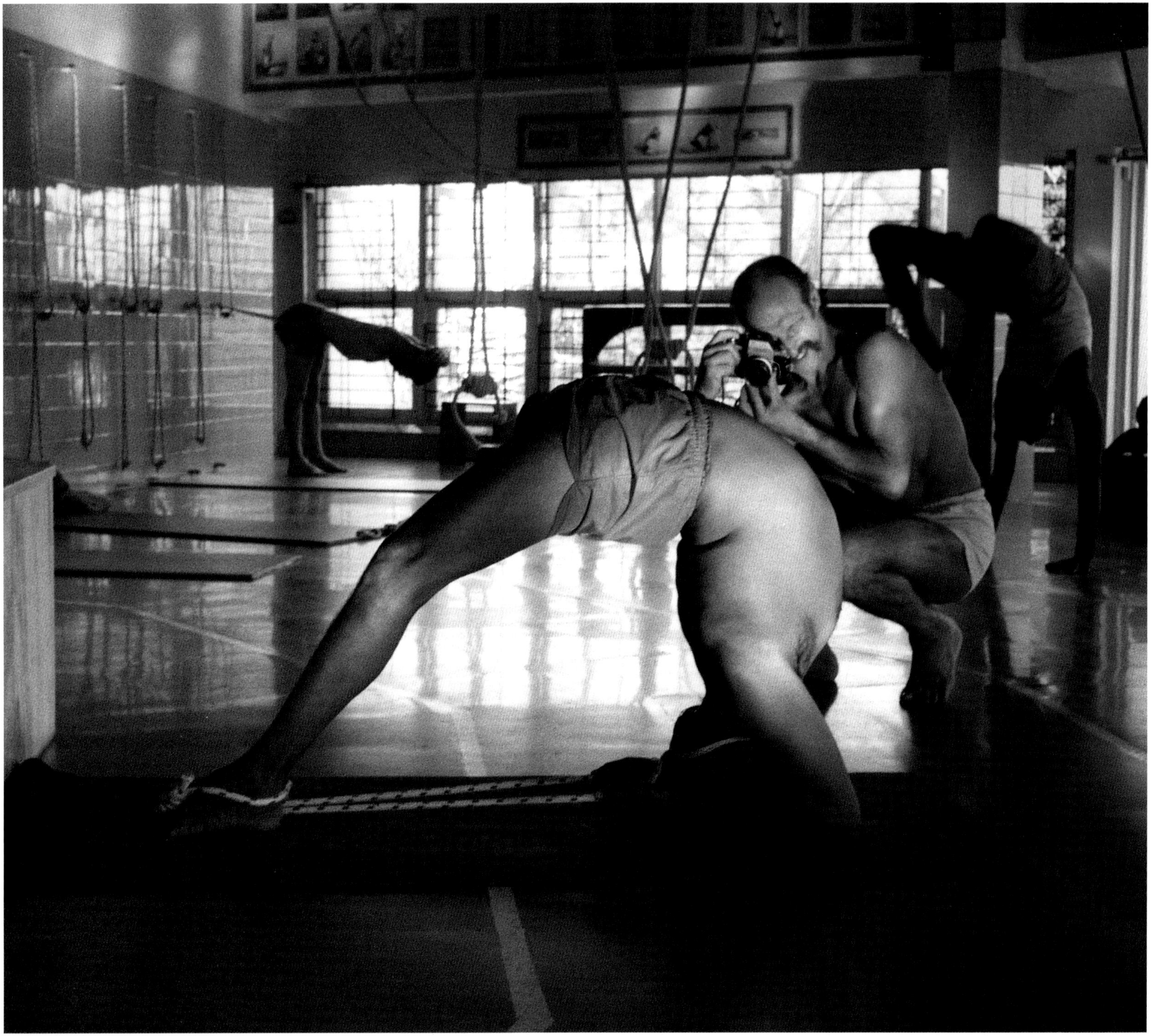

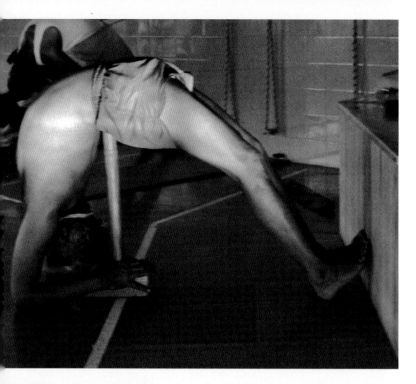

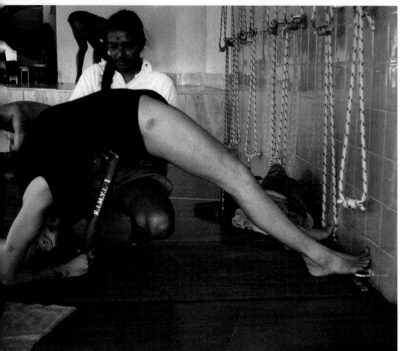

He told how he had got up in the very early hours to come in and practise, to make his body like one of the students that he had been working with. To understand how to teach them, he would make his body like theirs. This is the art of teaching.

PL

Many years ago, I was in Pune on an intensive, and standing on the steps of the *asana* hall observing a medical class in progress. Suddenly Guruji marched up to the steps, looked straight at me and said in a strict voice, "Are you just going to stand there or are you going to help?!" I had been teaching and was already qualified by him, but I consider that moment to be my real initiation into Iyengar yoga. Guruji was like a dynamo in the medical classes, everywhere at once. We would be running all over the hall trying to keep up with him. I wrote down all the sequences for the patients he told me to help. But if he did one thing one day, he would change it the next, ever in the moment according to the need of the patient. One day he said that he hadn't slept all night. When I asked him why, he said in order to find out how to help a particular patient he had tried to almost recreate his condition in himself and only then was he able understand. What compassion! He had the insight and touch of a healer par excellence.

AD

Classes in those days were unrelenting. Guruji's eyes and presence were everywhere. In his eyes we were rightly green novices, even if we may have been strong enough to deal with the physical load. He wanted more that that. He wanted absorption, total self-observation at all times. He demanded we surrender to him, and if we had doubts about something, he asked us to give over in class, and then review our doubts after the class. It was intense, it was exhilarating, and it was the most life-changing thing I had ever done. There was no looking back from that time in Pune. It was about practice and self reflection, and more practice and more self-questioning. There was no other way to do yoga with Guruji and it was transformational.

PL

What was it like to be around him in the early days? You never knew what he was going to do or say or if you would be called up. In those days he was really fierce. He was the Lion of Pune. The classes were much more doing, less reflection. So he would exhaust us, truly. We would sit on the bench outside the Institute thinking, "It's going to be really hard to walk home." But we loved it.

When Guruji was standing in front of us, we felt he could see or feel every thought we were having. That he could see right through us. He was incredibly savvy psychologically.

One day I was doing *Viparita Dandasana* and I was dropping back right near the wall. Guruji was very quiet, but I could feel him coming close. The first thing I thought was, I have to stabilise myself. He stood in front of me, put his hands on my feet, and took me into *Sirsapadasana*. And I thought I could never do that pose. When he adjusted me in that pose, I had to stabilise, but then I also surrendered. I had trust in myself and in him. That was how I really learned how to surrender. It was a transformative moment for me. I felt like I went into a deep part of my being. And he didn't take me out of it either. I had to figure out how to get out of it myself!

He brought something out in us that we couldn't bring out on our own.

PW

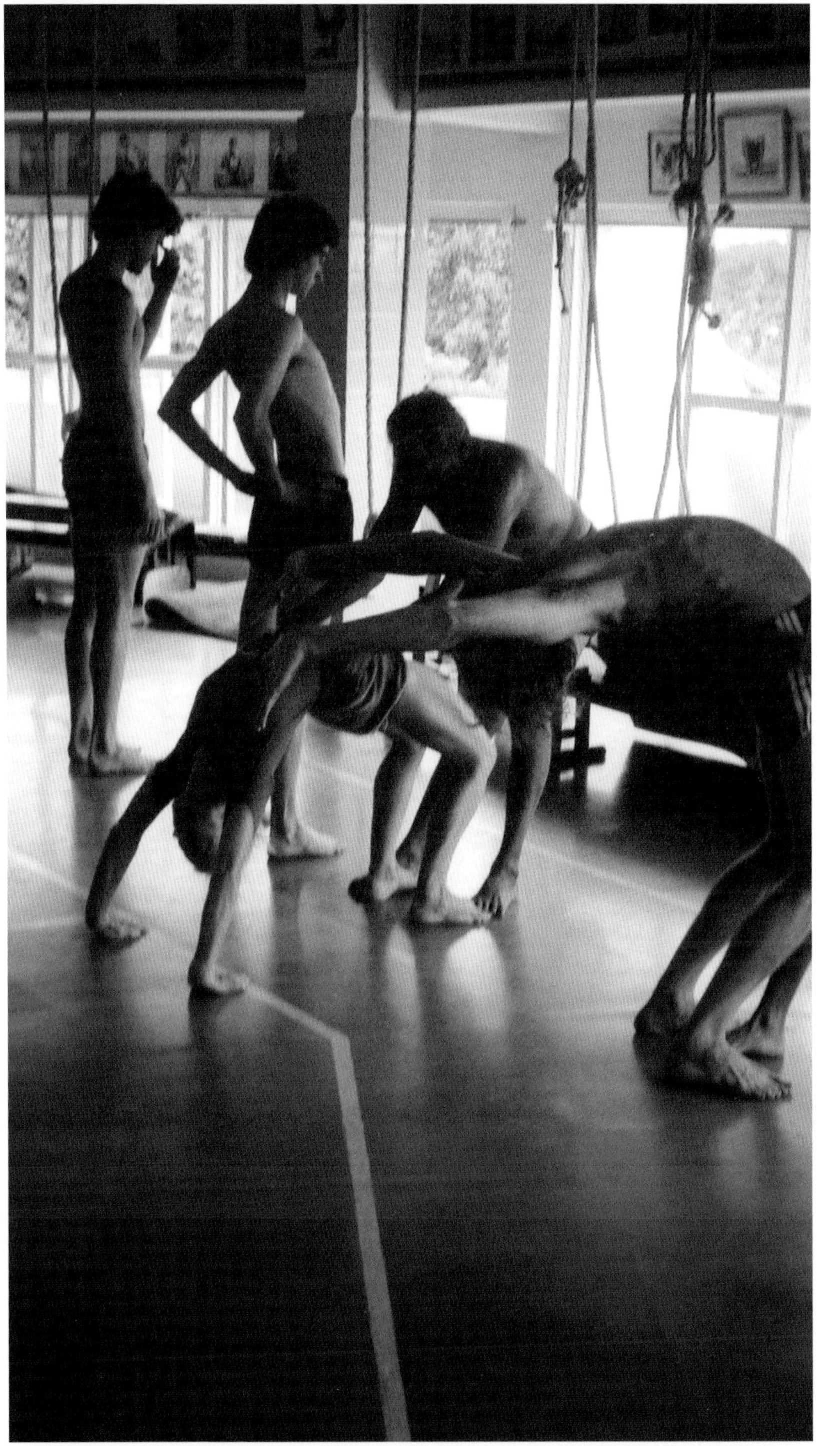
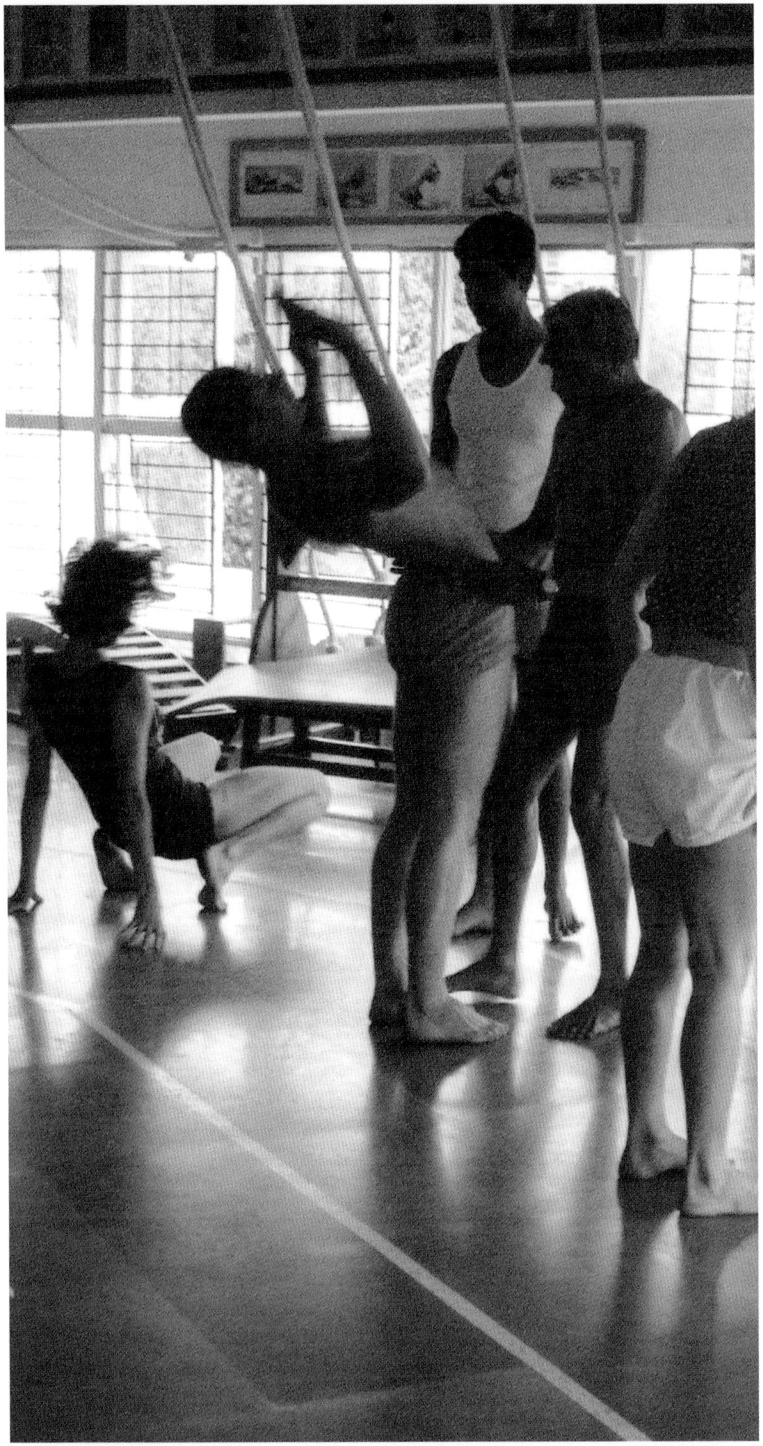

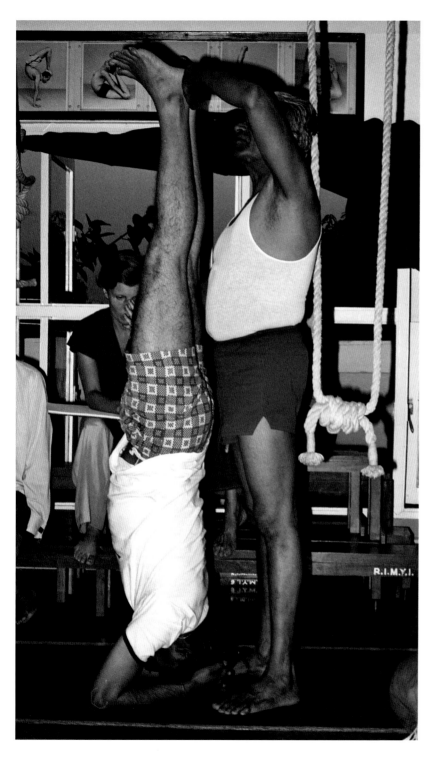

He used to stand in front of us when we were doing *Sirsasana* with our big toe on his forehead and then he adjusted the pose. That was really for me something about the greatness of this man because I knew he was an orthodox Brahmin. This great man was putting our feet on his head to correct our poses. This really impressed me.

My very first class with Guruji was an advanced class. He did headstand and we should follow in the class. I was a beginner in Iyengar yoga so I was not understanding the things that he was asking us to do. On my left was Shah and on my right was Pandu. Guruji said, "Hey Geeta, go and correct this French fellow. They think they know everything—they are gurus!" I said, "I am not a guru" and Shah whispered to me, "Shut up!" After the class I went to talk to Guruji and he was watching me intently. And I said the thing that nobody should have said to him at that time. I said, "I am very sorry, but I don't understand your English." He watched me very fiercely and brought his two fingertips just in front of my eyes and said, "But God gave you two eyes." The moment he said that, I prostrated and touched his feet. Then I lifted my head, his fierce eyes were suddenly so soft, and a deep affection was shining forth from their depths. I felt that I was in front of a very special soul and my heart was full of love. From that first moment I knew that he was my Guru.

FB (Faeq Biria)

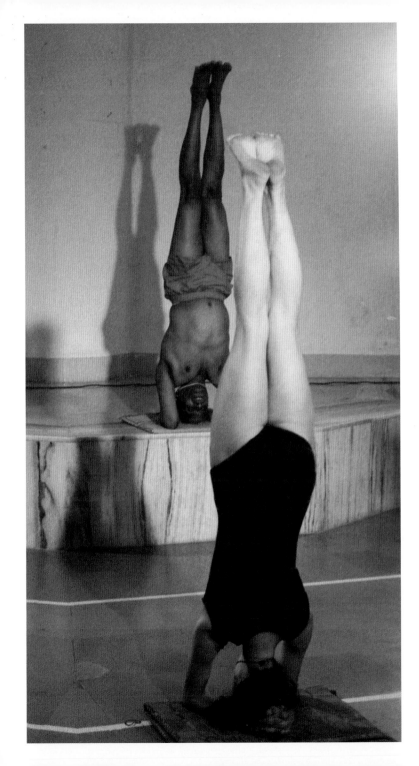

One day he was practising *Sirsasana* in the hall and a friend of mine and I were near him. Everyone always tried to be near him when he was practising. We were also doing our *Sirsasana* and he was doing his and he came down and we came down. He said, "Come here, come here." He said, "Look at the imprint of my head and elbows on the blanket. Put your head exactly where I put mine and do your *Sirsasana*." And it was like you floated away—it was the most amazing sensation. The way his weight must have been distributed and those marks of his arms and his head. I remember putting my head exactly where the imprint was. It was immediate plumb line alignment in my body. So light.

AD

After I had been practising over 10 years a friend of mine asked me to teach his classes while he was away for 3 months. Guruji said, "He's going away for 3 months, why don't you teach the classes?" I asked him if he thought I was capable of teaching, and he said yes, so I accepted the offer to teach. That is the difference. We follow the gurus' tradition of the *guru-shisya parampara* (succession of gurus and disciples in traditional Vedic culture). Which means that unless the teacher gives you permission to teach, you do not teach.

JB (Jawahar Bangera)

One day when I was 15 years old, Guruji and Geetaji came for the children's class. I was playing around before the class and they called over to me to talk to them. I was scared I was going to get in trouble as we were supposed to be practising. They told me to go on the stage and start teaching the class. I was shocked. I said I don't know how to teach. I was quite scared. They said go ahead. Geetaji said, "I have also been a teacher from my childhood. I had to learn and you also have to learn! Go up on the stage and start teaching." So my teaching started just like that. We never decided that we wanted to be yoga teachers, it just happened.

AJ (Abhay Javakhedkar)

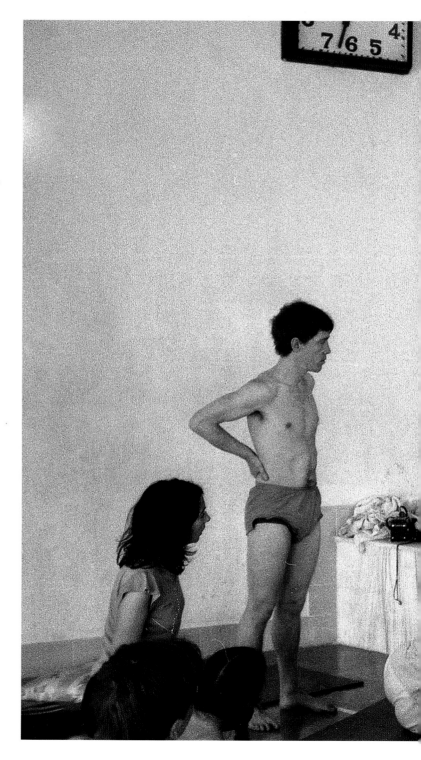

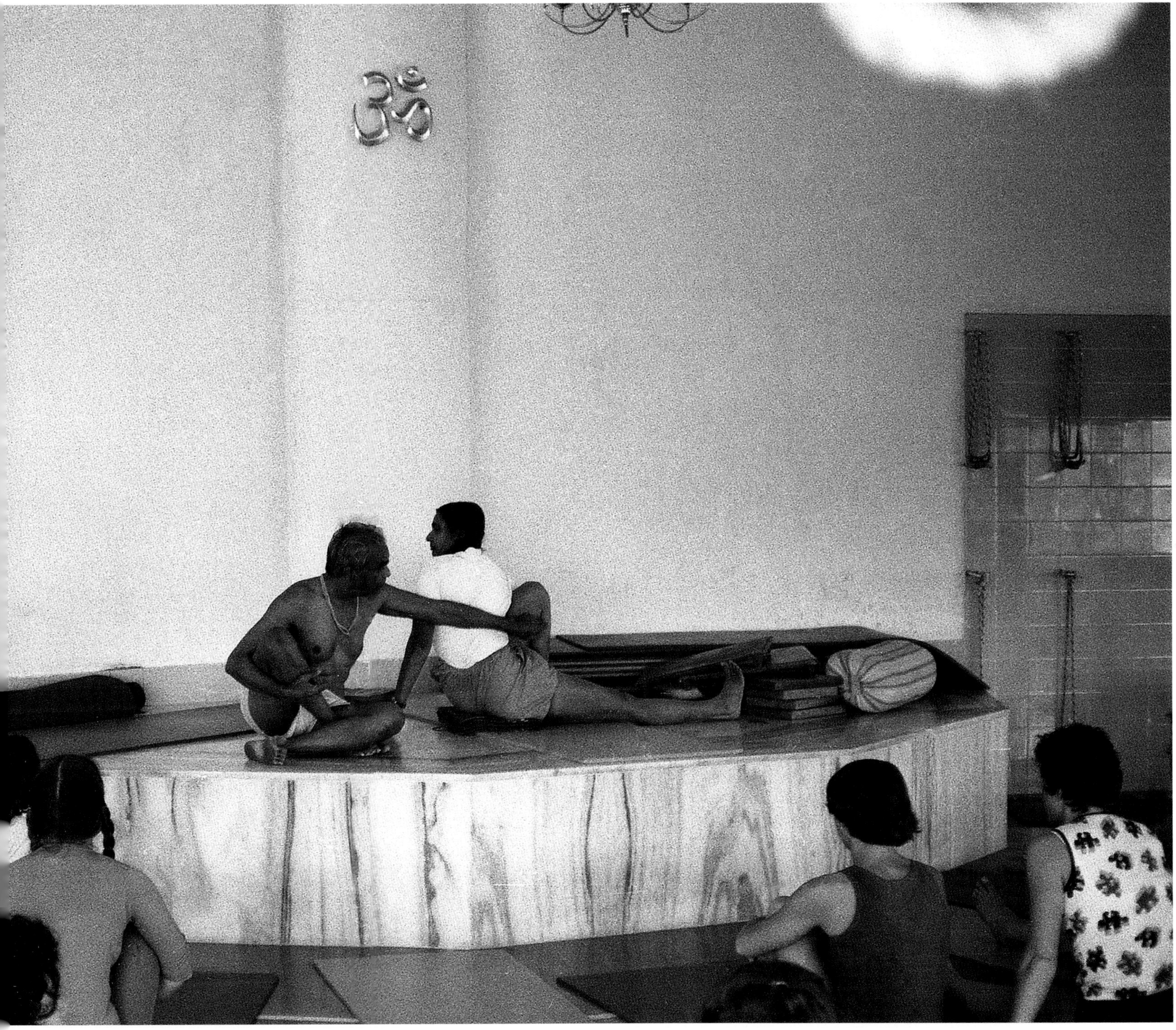

Especially on backbending days you could see the intensity in his eyes. He was all charged—the battery was full. You dare not look into his eyes. We all had to make an assembly line for the dropbacks. He would catch each one and drop you back. By the time we recovered and were back on our feet he was already back at the top of the line waiting for us.

NK

The classes in Pune in 1976 were some of the hardest classes I remember. He would push us harder and harder and harder. One morning we had class at 7 a.m. and many of us were there a few minutes early. He asked the man who was working for the Institute as the rickshaw driver to come up and immediately made him do *Mandalasana* extolling the fact that this man who was not a yogi could be made to do this pose without any warm ups. The next thing we knew he was telling us to do headstand drop backs with no warm-ups; no nothing. He wanted six of each and then for us to go on and do more backbends culminating in *Mandalasana*. For starters I had never done a headstand drop back so I was trying to go slowly as I was worried about my back. He saw me and rushed over and said ,"What are you waiting for?" He just pushed me over into the drop back and said, "Accept your failures and move on." After that I just seemed to magically be able to do drop backs from *Sirsasana*.

JW

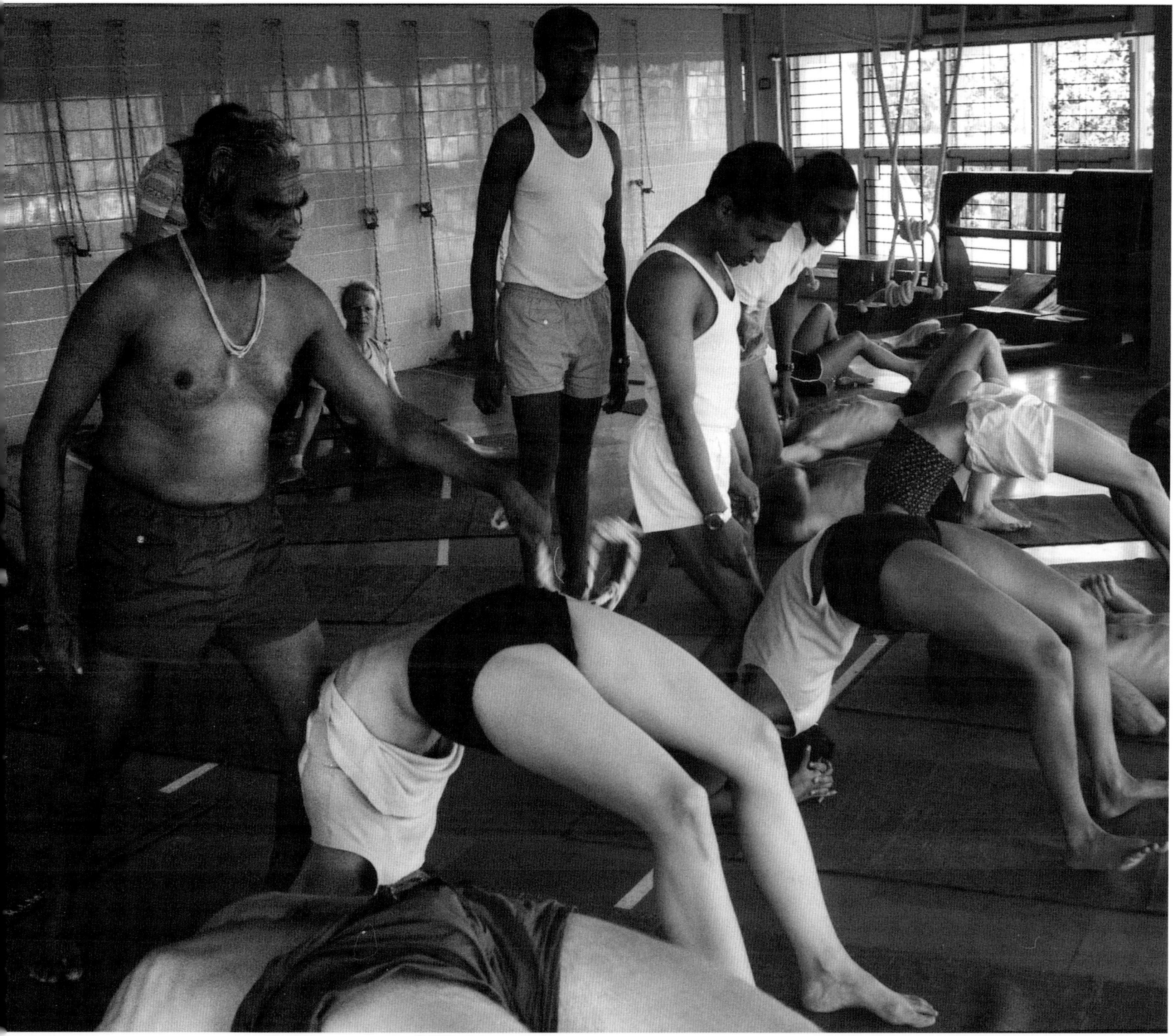

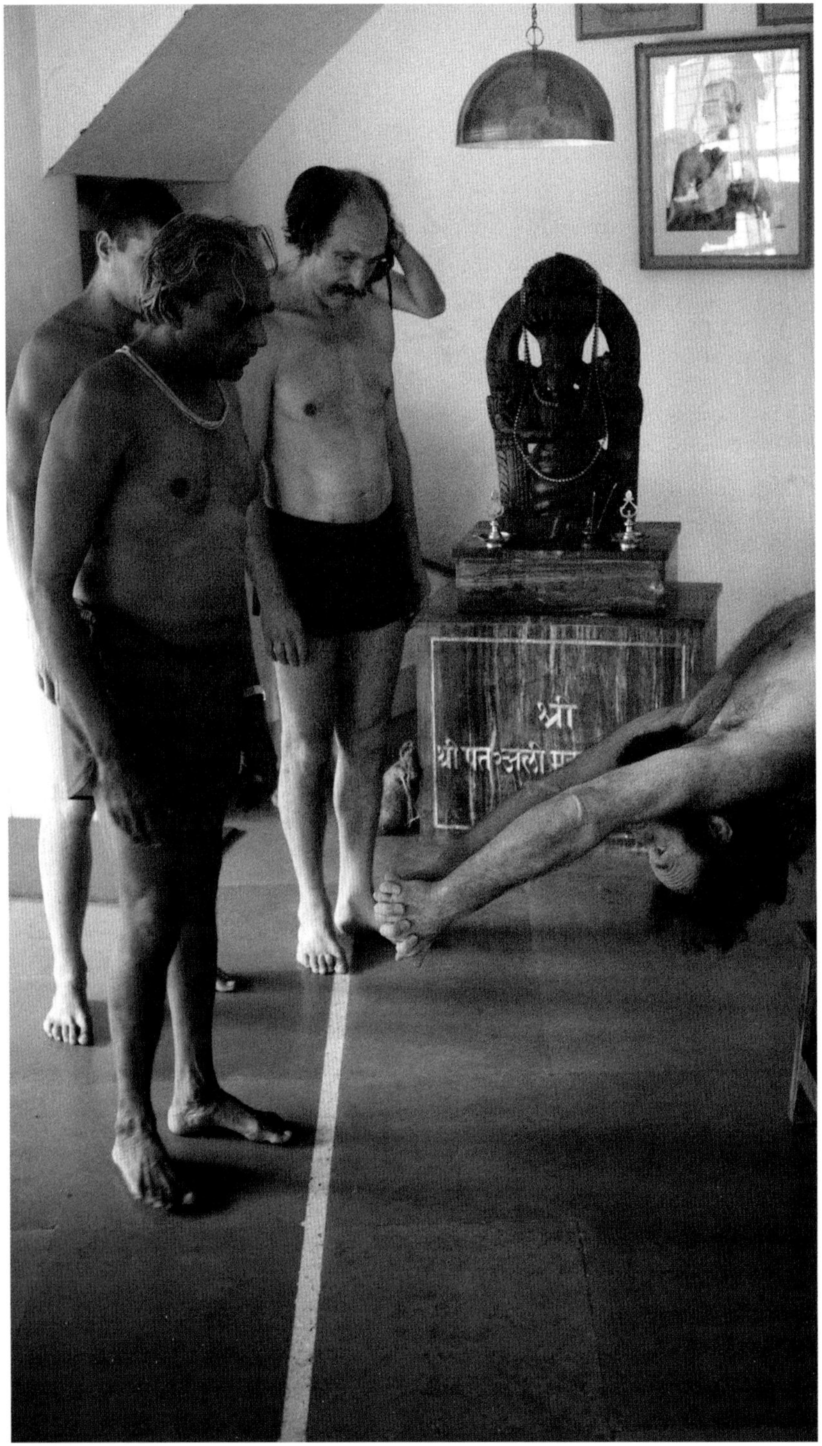
श्री

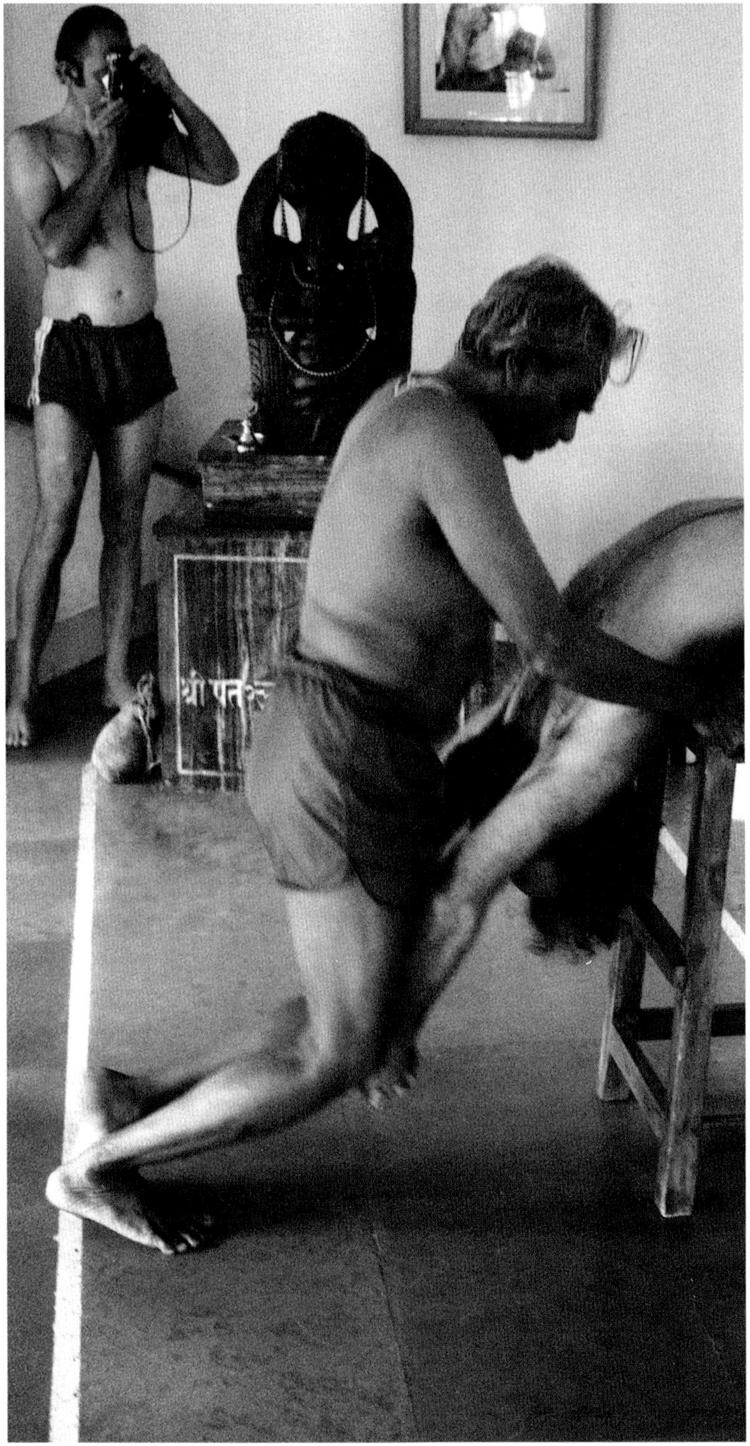

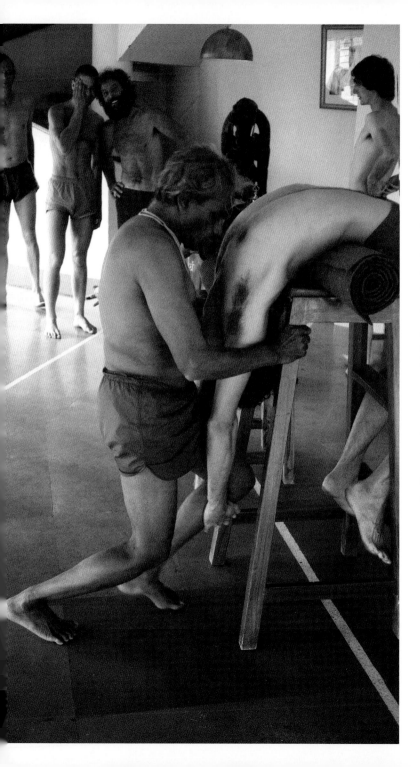

Guruji often gave strong, intense adjustments, quite quickly tempered by a fleeting smile that you might not even catch. His extraordinary adjustments often took you by surprise. The way it worked best was to completely surrender. You would then find yourself more deeply in a pose than you had ever achieved yourself. Yet even in these moments he might show his unexpected sense of humour in the midst of his ferocity.

His intention was to teach you, or to use you to teach something to the class. It was always about the yoga, about you 'getting it', and he stopped at nothing to make a point. In the old days of less modern props, and especially when he travelled, he would use a pencil, or a spoon, or a book behind your shoulder blades, or under your trapezius for example in *Sarvangasana* to get extra lift. He would use anything that came to hand to help sharpen your awareness. His hands, his feet, his head, everything was a tool. He seemed to grow extra limbs and strength for that very purpose.

He never forgot anything about any of his students. He seemed to have a visual memory of everything you had ever done in front of him.

PL

I still remember very clearly the first time I saw Guruji. I was very young and I was sent actually by my first teacher, Father Joe Pereira. He had an accident and he asked me to teach his class. Father Joe said, "Go to Guruji and learn with him and you will be able to teach my class." So very obediently I landed in the class with a note from Father Joe saying that he was in hospital and he asked me to join Guruji's class. He said, "OK!" So that's how I started my first day, that's how I started with him. I knew nothing about who he was.

When Father Joe was back teaching a few months later I stopped going to Guruji's classes. Father Joe noticed I wasn't in the class and he said I must go back. I went back to Guruji's class and I got this piercing look from him and he said, "I know her. She stopped coming. She didn't tell me." I asked if I could join again. He said, "Only if you are going to be regular."

He started that class with *Viparita Chakrasana*; *Urdhva Dhanurasana* with the feet on the platform and you jump. This was the first class I joined after my break. He remembered that I stopped suddenly. I have these vivid memories of how he started that class and how he made us to jump from the platform and then the whole class went on with at least 60 to 70 backbends in total with 10 *Viparita Chakrasanas* from the platform. Then we did jumping from the wall, then *Urdhva Dhanurasana*. You do your *Urdhva Dhanurasana*, then put your feet up on the wall. You walk up the wall and come over. So that's again *Viparita Chakrasana*, because at that time we couldn't do it in the middle of the room anyways. And all this while he was doing it in the middle of the room. So if we did 50 then he must have done a hundred. That's when his

dynamism hit me totally. That's when I decided in my head I'm going to die but do this time. There was no question of leaving or going away. All these imprints are still very vivid.

My love for philosophy grew after I started with yoga. I didn't know anything about yoga philosophy. But as I found myself to be so intrigued by yoga, I found changes taking place in my own self that I felt I wanted to know more about the philosophy behind it. The first book was *Light on Yoga*, followed by other books on yoga. That induced me to take philosophy as my major area of learning. So in a large way Guruji was instrumental in shaping my entire life after the age of 20.

FAR

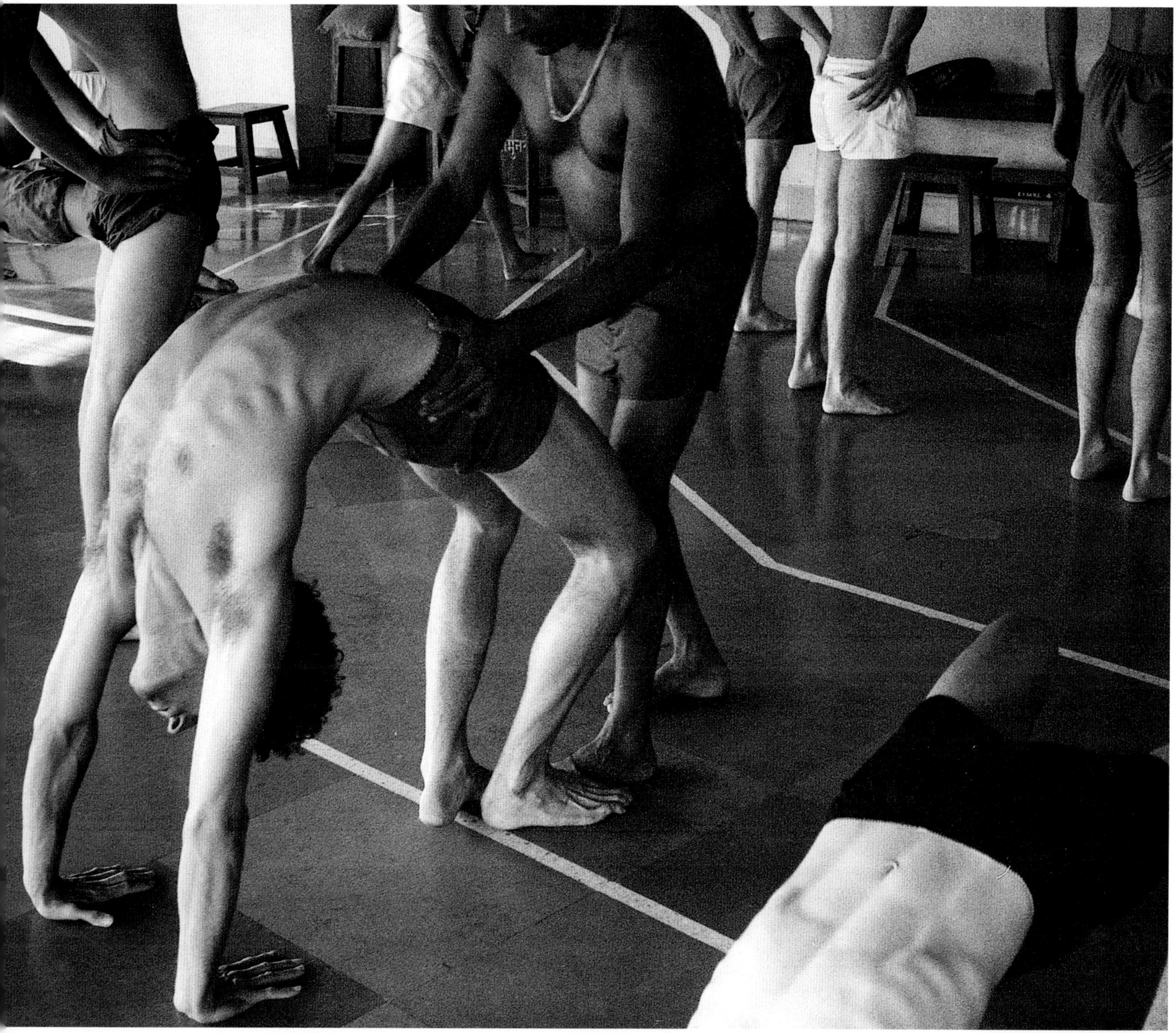

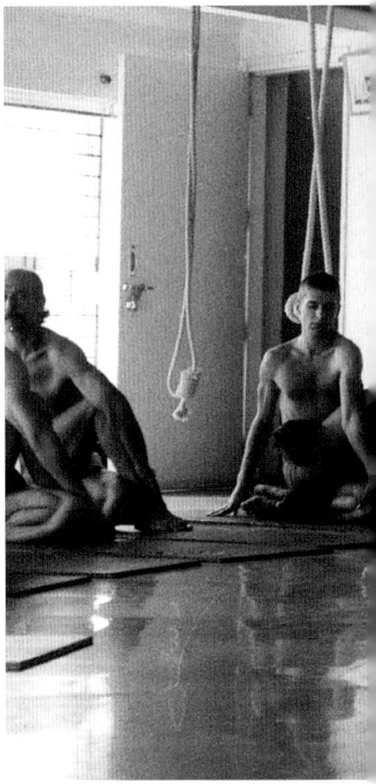
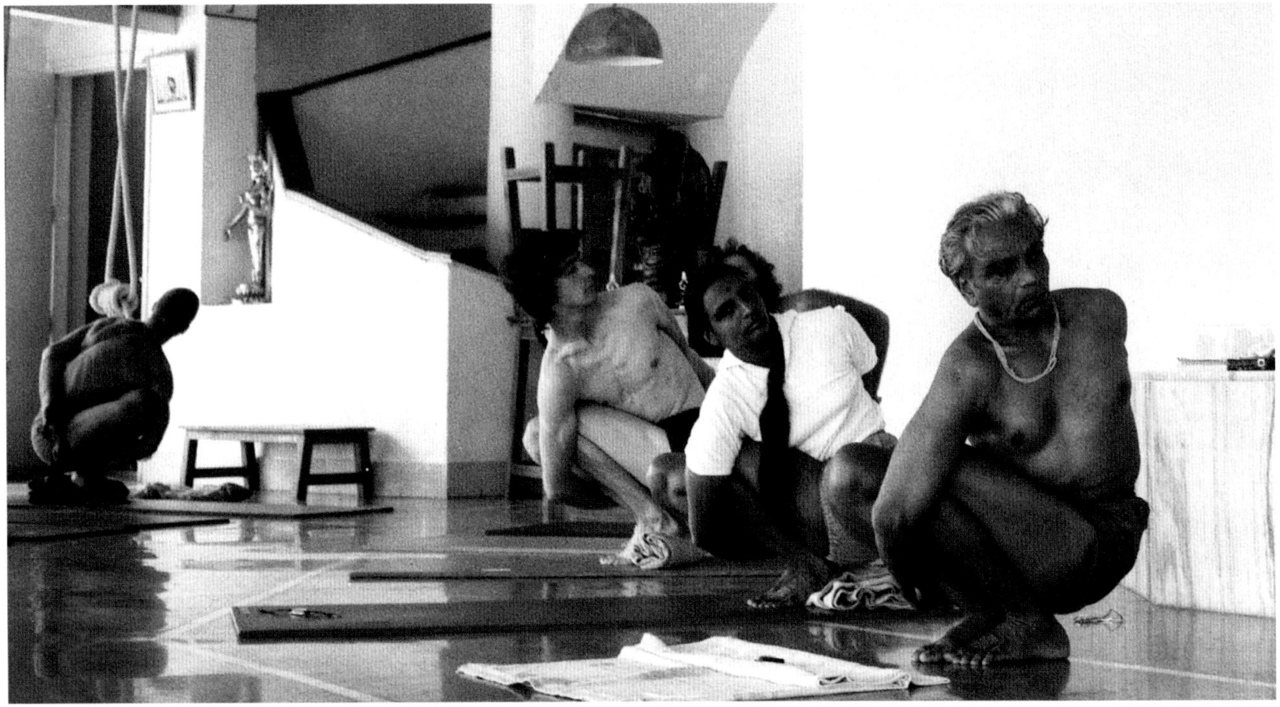
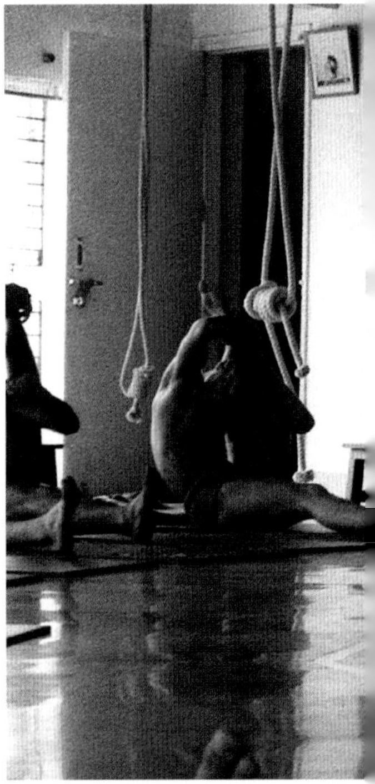
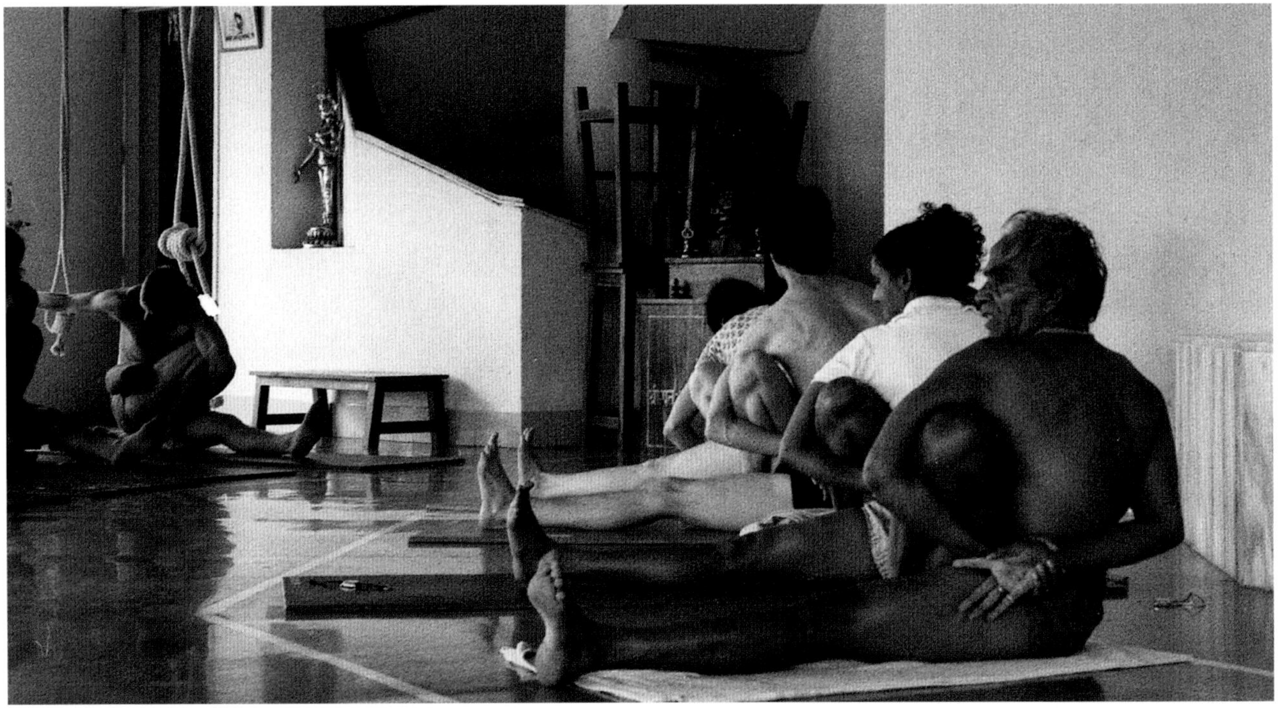

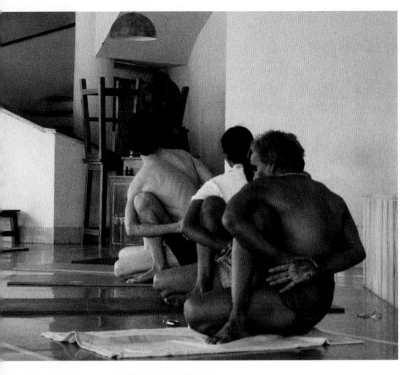

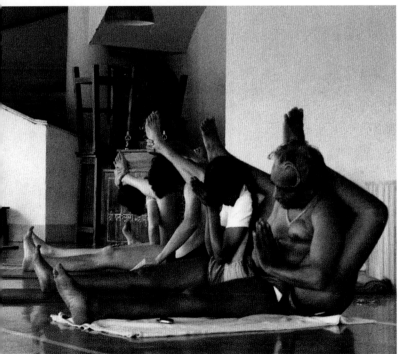

Imagine the challenge of holding poses next to Guruji as he led us in a small circle, or when he would jump up into full arm balance beside you and question why you were unable to maintain the pose correctly, "to the maximum!"

One week there were only eight of us and we had the privilege of practising with the Iyengars and Shah. I well remember the 15 minute *Paschimottanasana* and the long cool inversions.

AC

We used to spend Tuesday mornings doing forward bends, and the class was done mostly in silence with Guruji practising too.

Once when we were practising *Ardha Matsyendrasana,* I was a little confused and turned to the wrong side. He marched up to me and bellowed, "Do you want to teach the class? Why don't you go up there and teach the class?" I realised the worst thing I could have done was to have replied with any self-justification or apology, which could have invited more criticism so I decided to make my eyes as soft as I could. I saw Guruji looking into my eyes and he must have seen what I was trying to do, grunted and walked off, apparently satisfied or mollified.

RAW

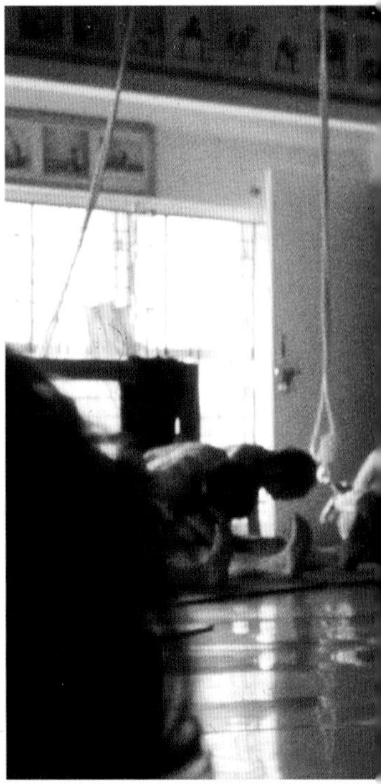
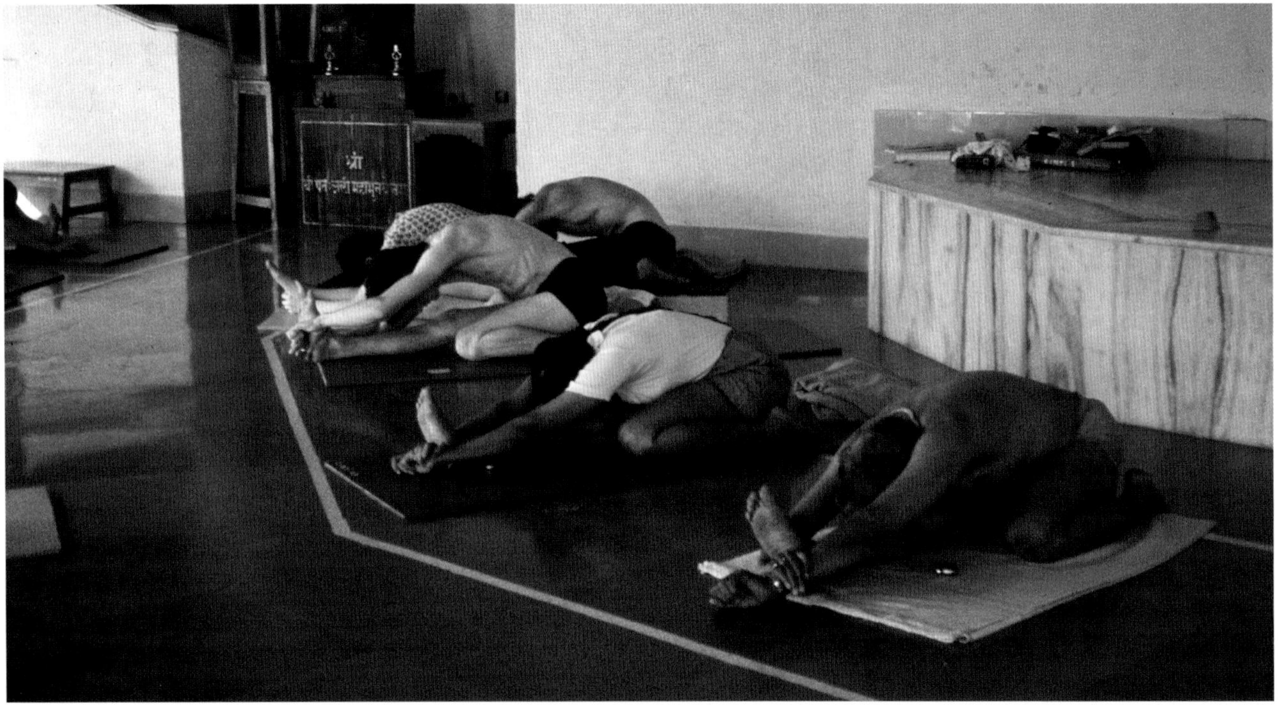
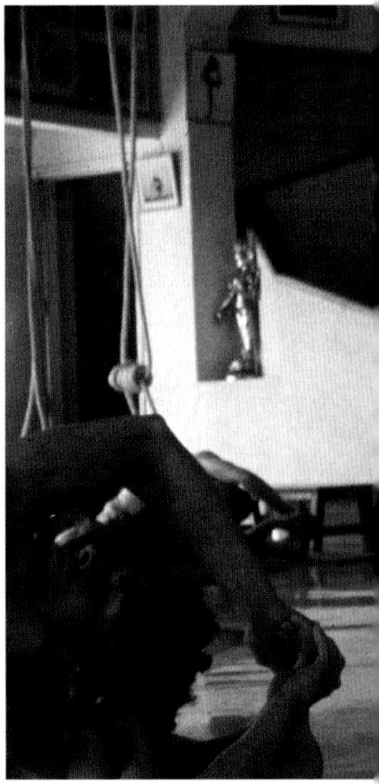
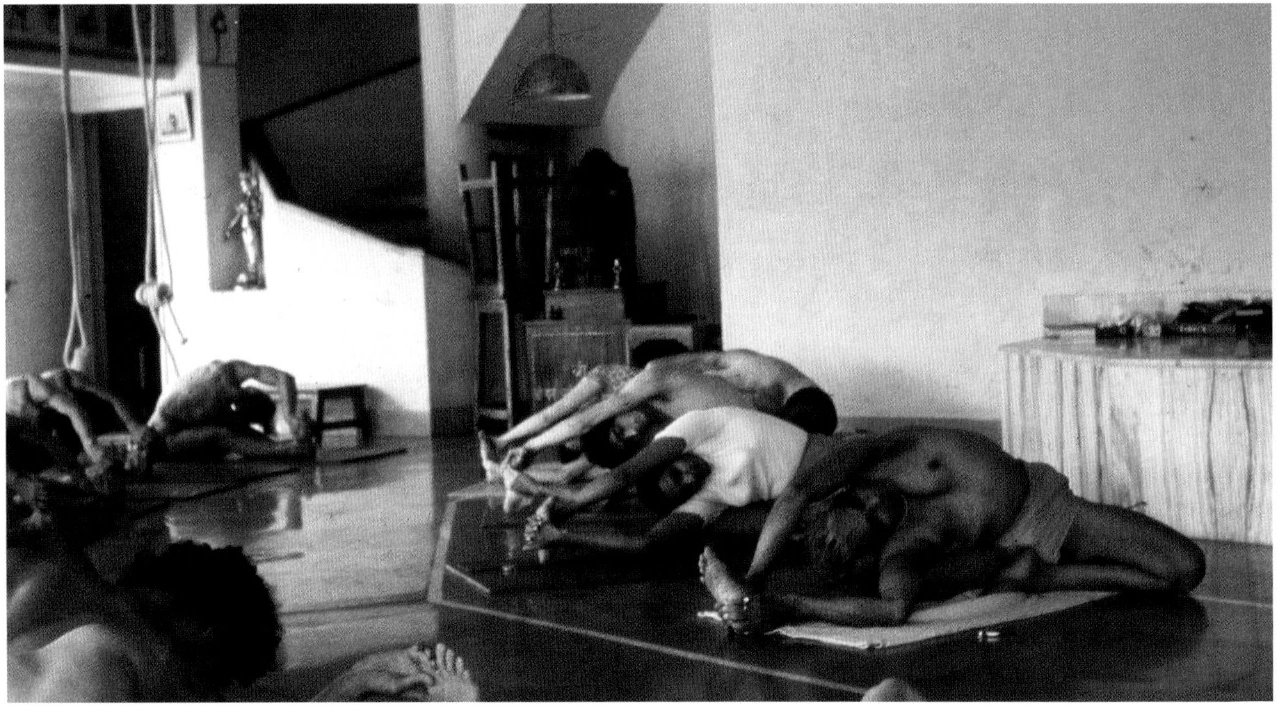

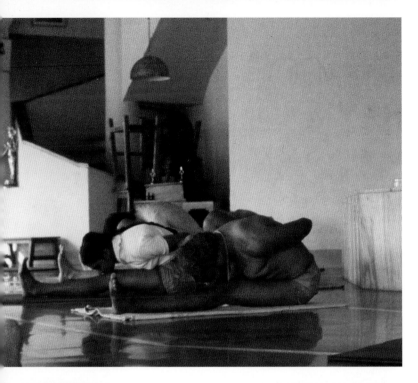

If you were doing forward bends, then he would actually come use his knees by the sides of our chest and then push us forward. So that is how he would do that. Even in *Paschimottanasana* he would stand on us then he would go to the next person and the third person.

BM

Seated forward extensions were something else again. We held each pose for at least five minutes, and often longer. I have a memory of lines of students with the head down in *Paschimottanasana* and Guruji walking from body to body as if he were walking across a river on stepping-stones. As he came to each back, before putting his full weight on it, he tested it with one foot (the other still on the body behind) to see if it would surrender to his full weight. We became so still and quiet after those forward bend classes. You could have heard a pin drop.

BC

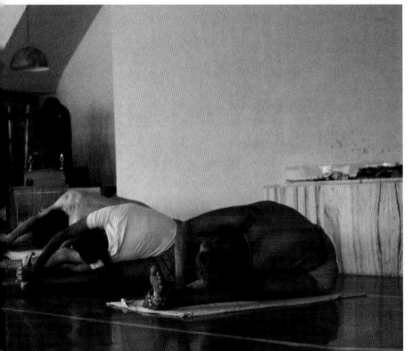

One unforgettable evening I was in class doing *Paschimottanasana*—unwittingly right underneath the ceiling ropes. I still remember seeing stars after he silently grabbed the rope and stood on my back—for a long time. However, the change to my *Paschimottanasana* was most impressive according to my friend next to me.

JP

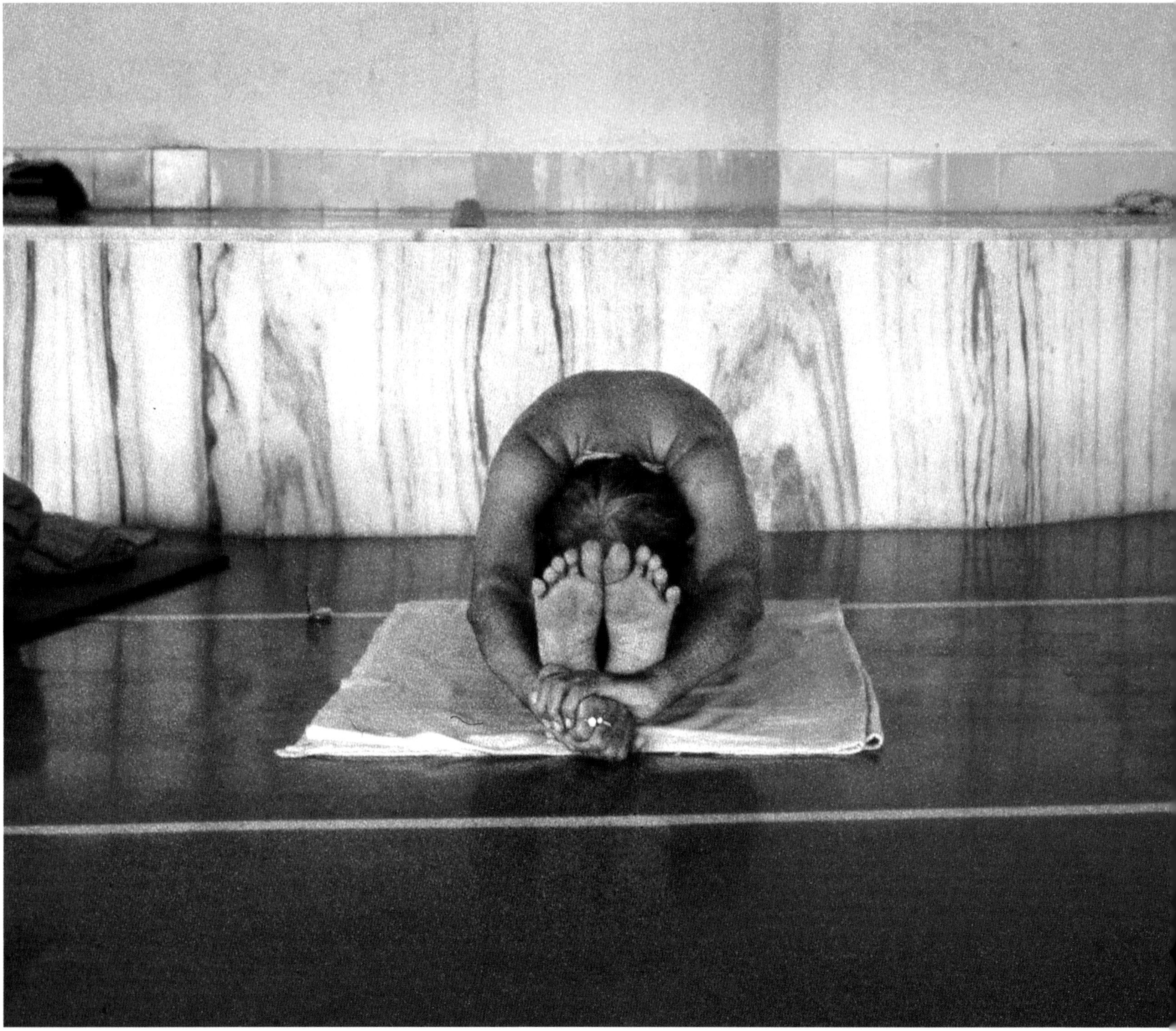

In the practice we stayed a long time in the poses. Once he put me in *Paschimottanasana* and put on the weight and after half an hour he was still not coming. Then he came and lifted the weight off. And I thought, "This is my last day of yoga." That pain—what I had to bear. I thought, "From tomorrow onwards I'm not coming." I felt I had decided and, "This was enough." And after half an hour he came and lifted the weights. The weights were very heavy—up to 100 lbs. You cannot get up with those heavy weights on you. After half an hour with the heavy weights I came half way up. You cannot come immediately straight up after that. And I said, "I'm not leaving yoga in my life!"

When I came up, I felt, "Oh, yoga is this." While I was there with the weights on in the pose, pain was there, but when I came up, something totally different was there. The whole day I was realising that something was different for me. I said "Wow, this is yoga!"

VD

The *Paschimottanasana* was so strong. After the class I was weeping. It was so intense. I wasn't crying because it was intense, I was crying because something in my body was understanding something. I realised how opened I felt. I felt like I'd been woken up. It was an amazing feeling. It was such a strong experience—like facing myself. Feeling all of my ineptitudes and working with it. I was right there focused and working with it. I was facing what was going on in my mind and my body in the present.

CC

One evening we came to the class to find, with virtually no notice to Guruji, that a film crew was there to film the class. Guruji organised us in rows and taught a very intense class where he was on the stage demonstrating, as well as adjusting the students and sometimes on the floor next to us doing the poses. He wanted to maximise yoga's exposure to the world and gave freely to all who would help him share.

JP

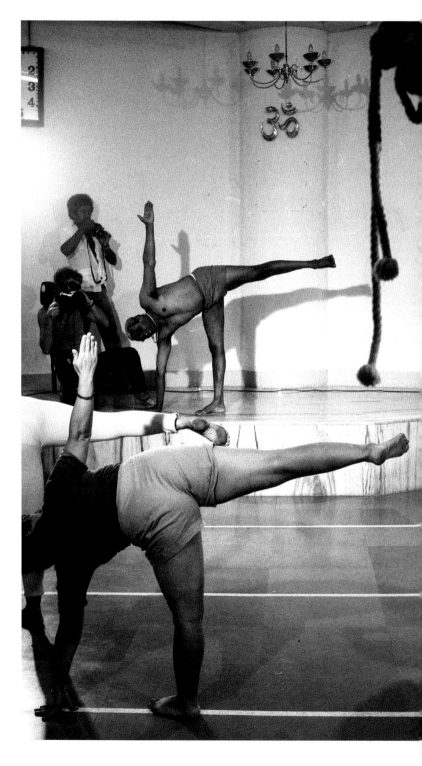

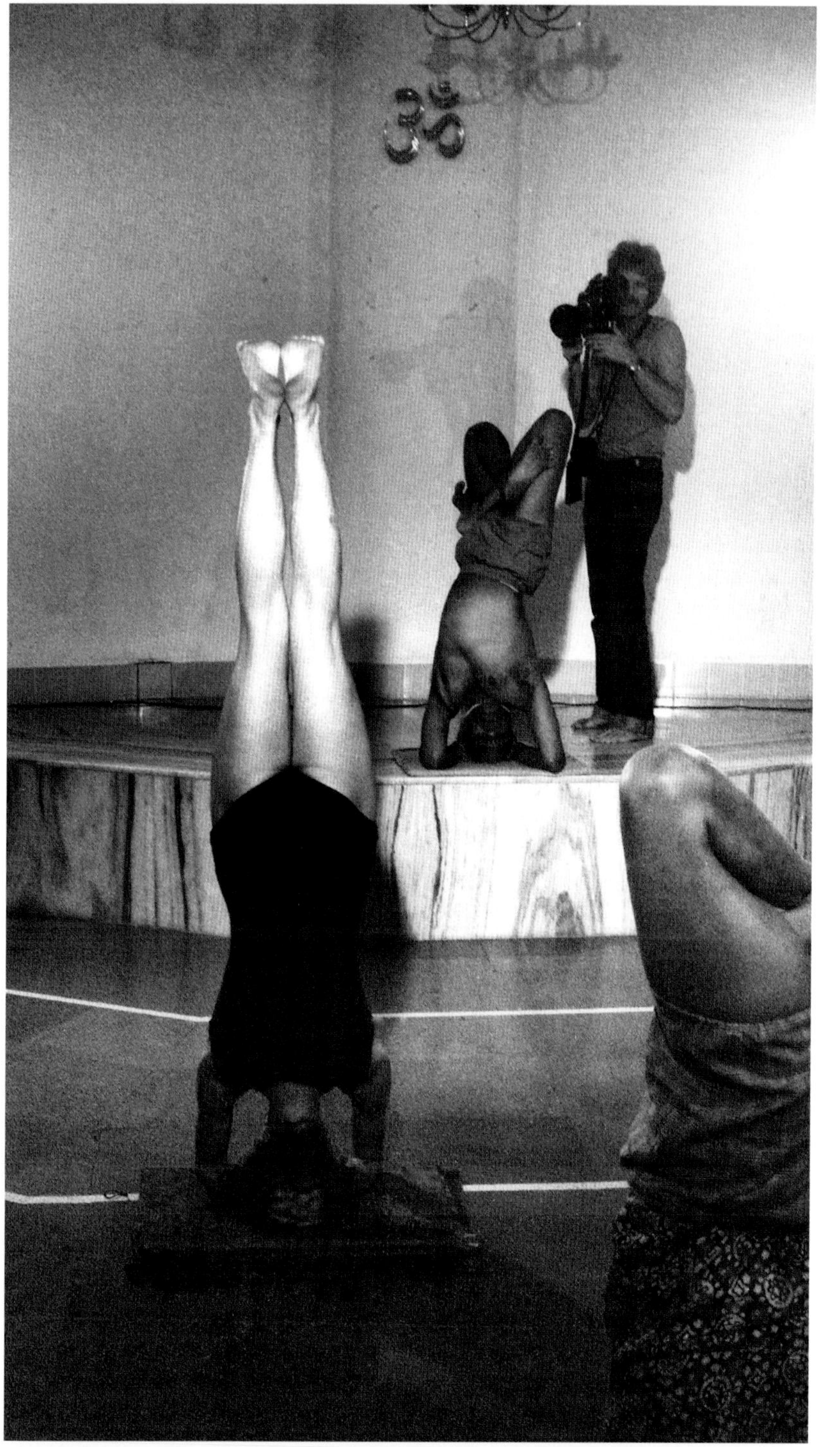

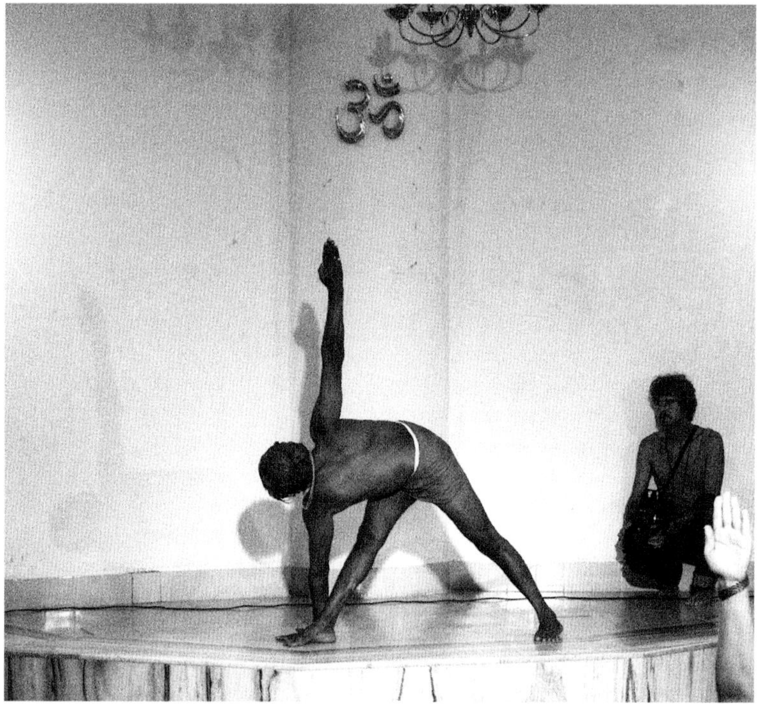

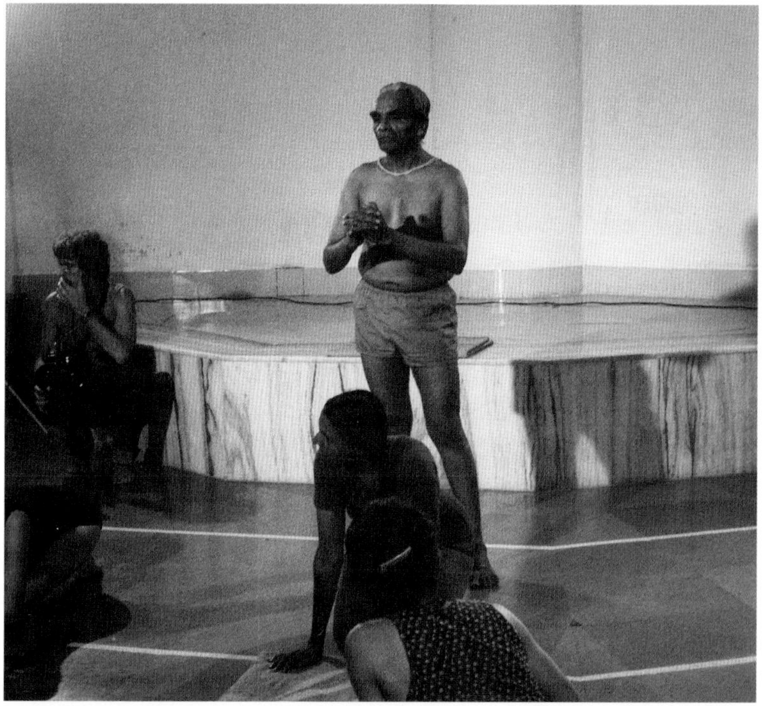

Guruji would walk to the other side of the hall during a class. He gave us an instruction for a variation in *Sirsasana*. Without looking, he called out to a student, "Why are you bending your knees?" He had eyes in the back of his head! He always knew what you were doing, even without actually looking. After that no one eased off their intense application even for a minute, no matter where he was.

He brought me on stage for *Parsvotttanasana*—he then turned to the group and said this was how not to do the pose... He said I was only doing with pride. I felt I was trying hard for the Master. He had no patience with people doing an *asana* in that sort of external way. You had to do it for the sake of yoga. He was uninterested in our 'trying'—"Don't try, just do," he would often say. He was intolerant of our pride, of our wanting to please.

He gave me an open handed slap on the thigh in a standing pose when I wasn't following his instruction for the legs. He then smiled and said, "Now you will remember that point, where the imprint is." I never forgot it, but it was also evident he had a purpose behind each admonishment. It never seemed personal. It was about creating sharpness and bringing some intelligence to each pose.

He was untiring in his efforts and enthusiasm. He corrected all of us, constantly, with his own hands.

PL

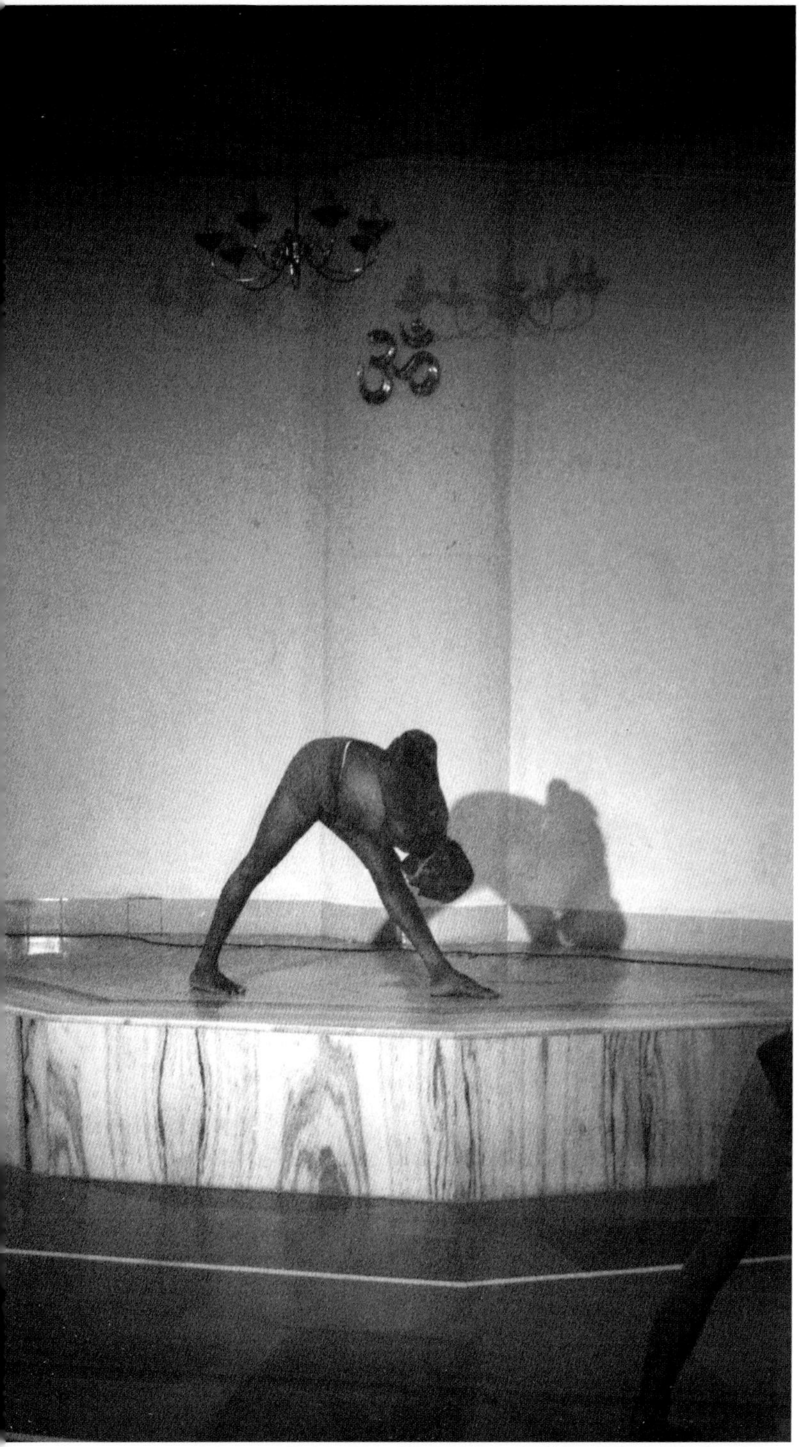
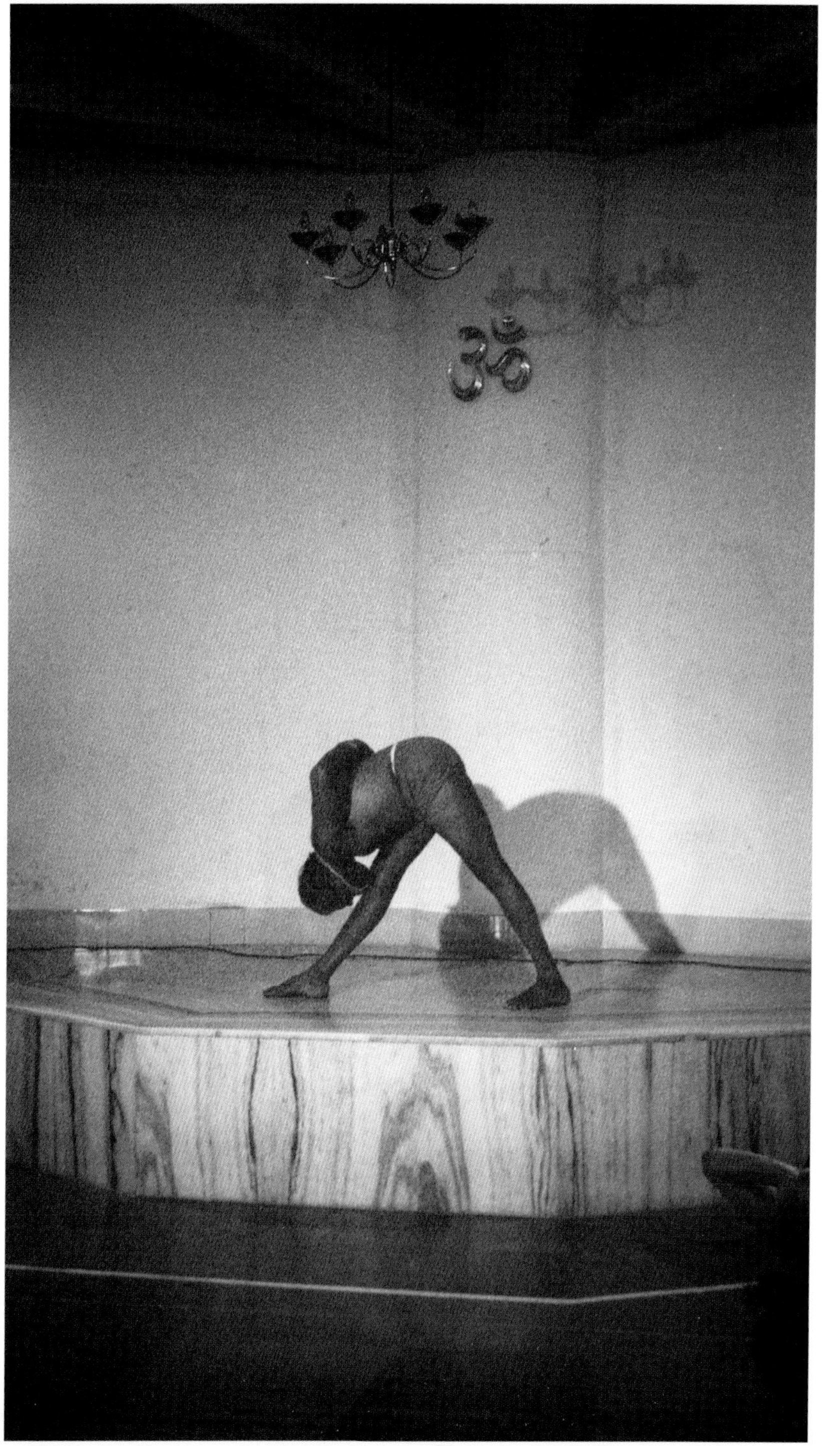

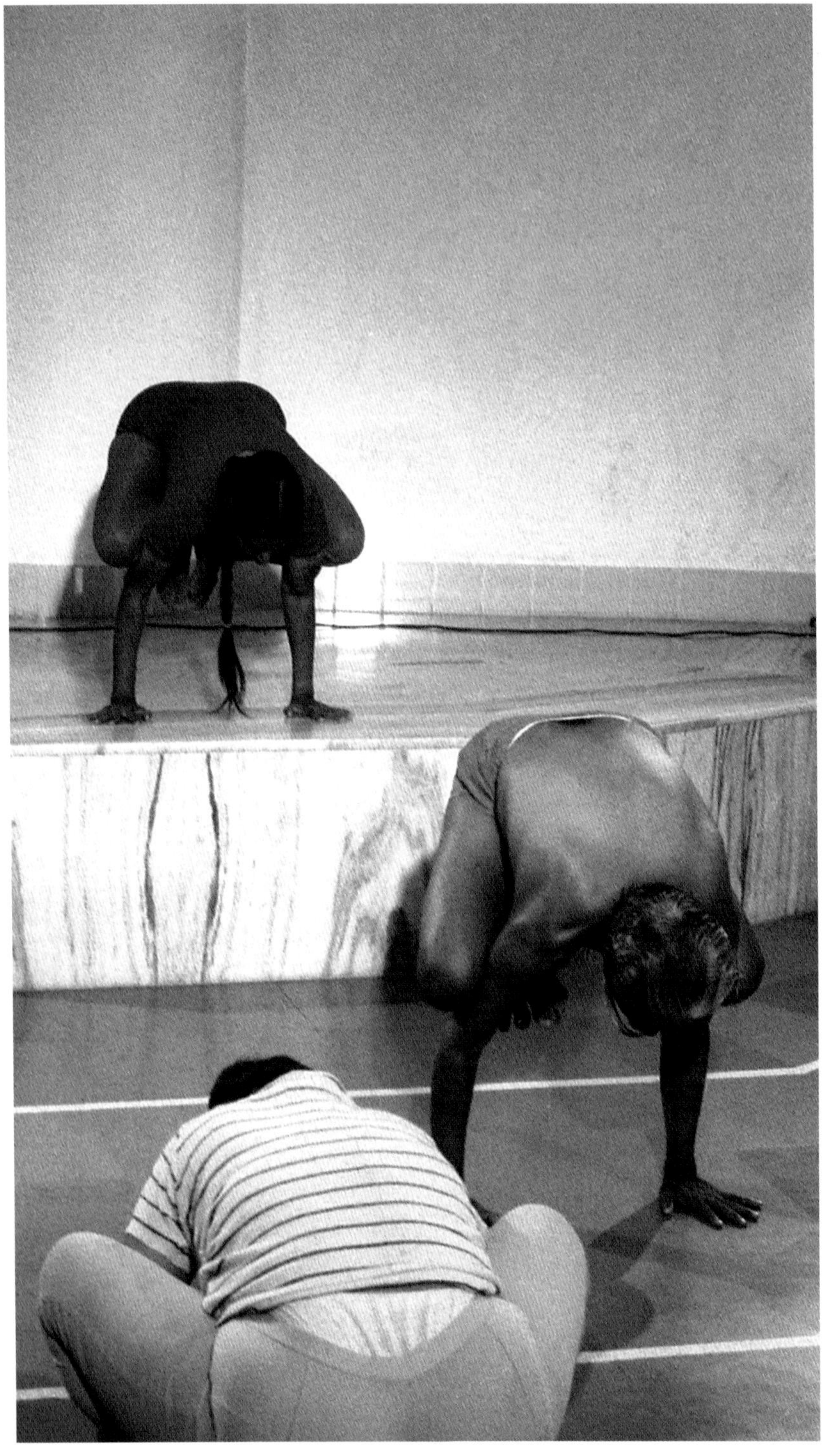
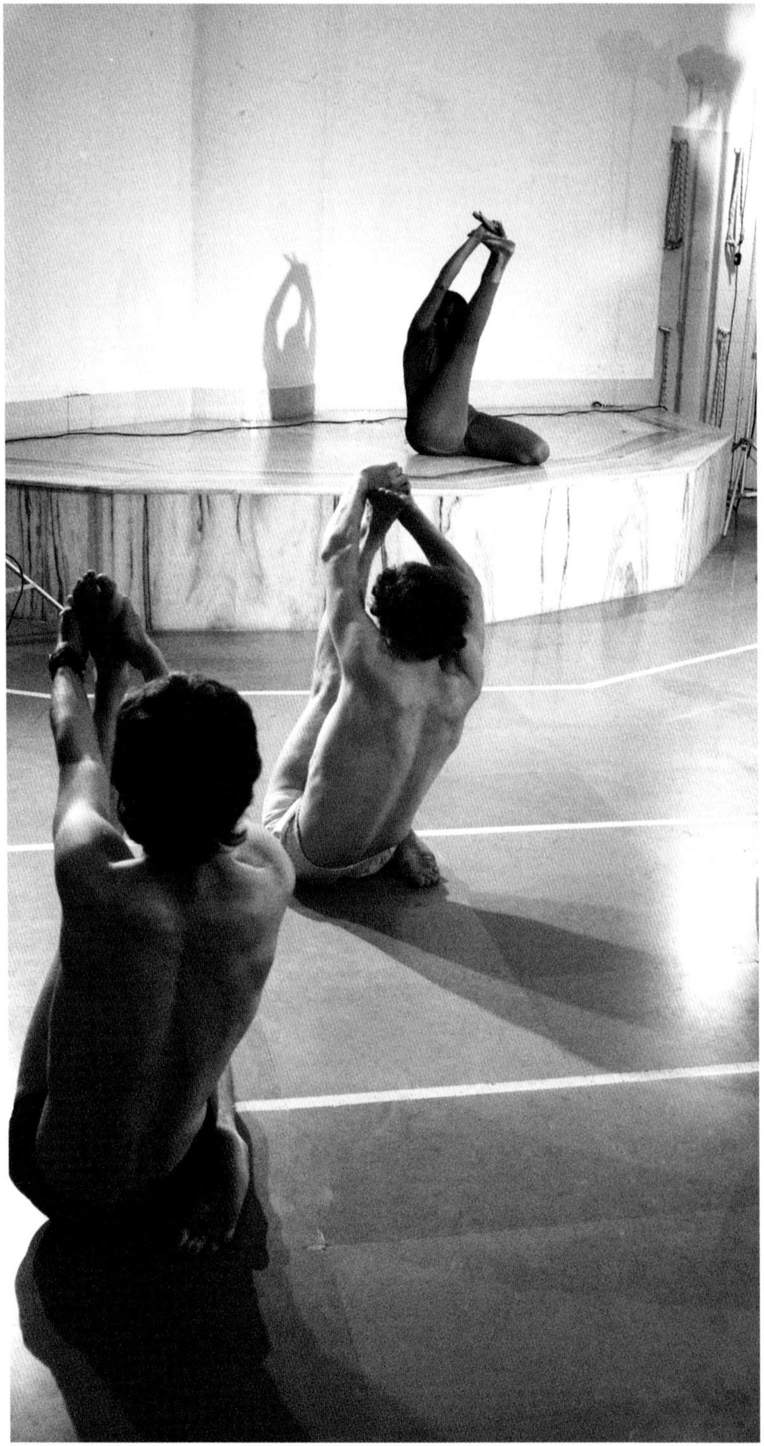

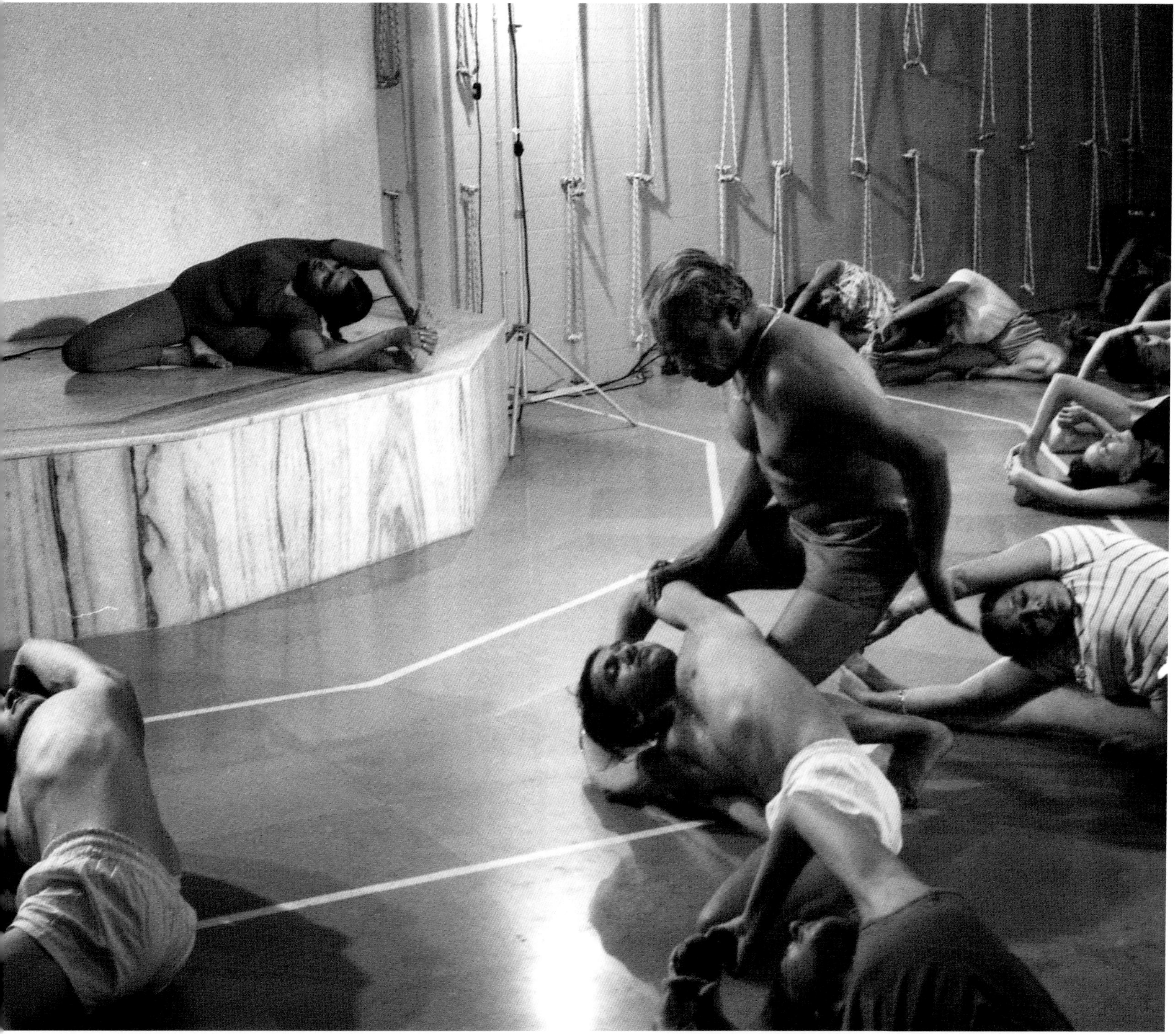

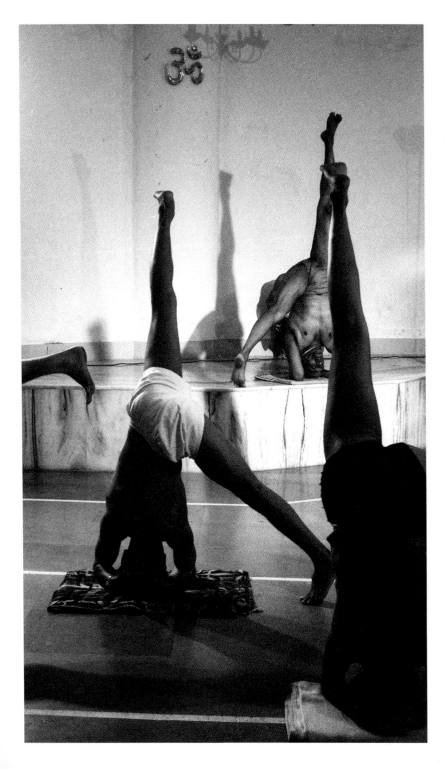

Guruji did not only teach with his words, demonstrations and actions but something far beyond. It was quite surprising that if he walked around you, your *asana* just changed without him saying anything—even when you were not aware that he was around you. If he was standing near you—you could stay in an *asana* endlessly. As a youngster, I thought that it was will-power and fear that made us stay. But today, I realise that he could communicate with my body, my mind and consciousness more that I myself could. Unknown to myself, I was getting introduced to the subject of yoga.

RM (Rajvi Mehta)

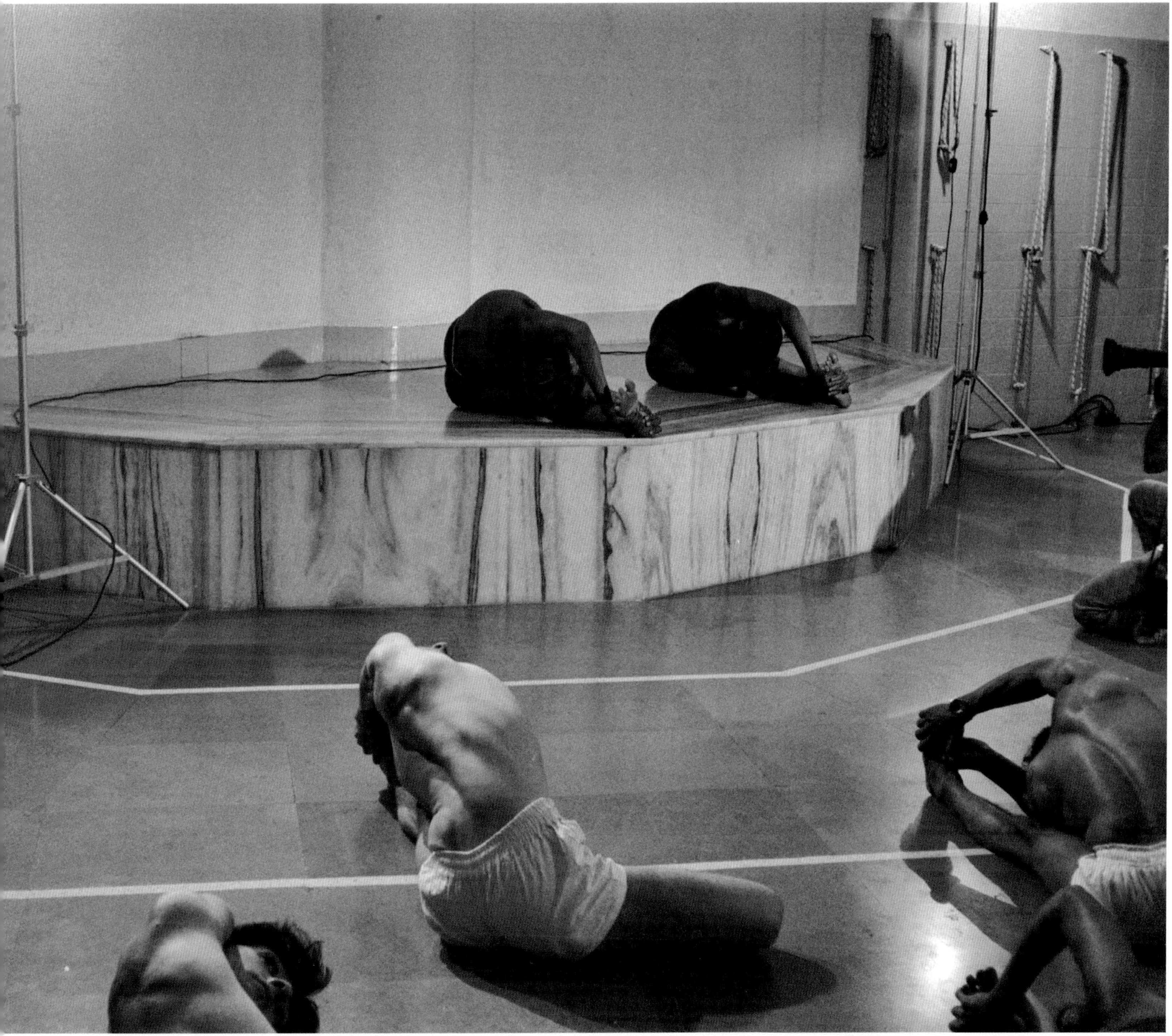

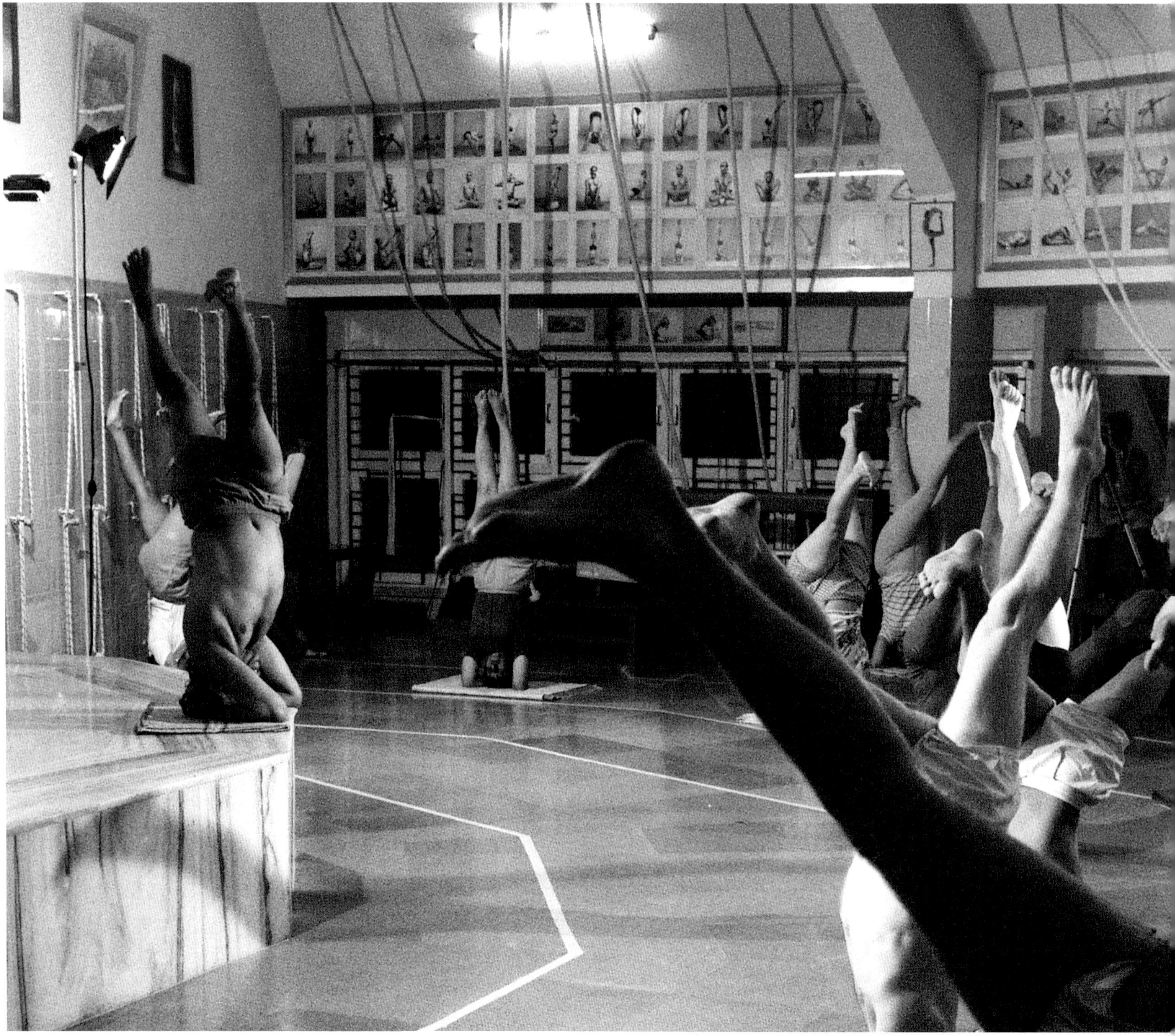

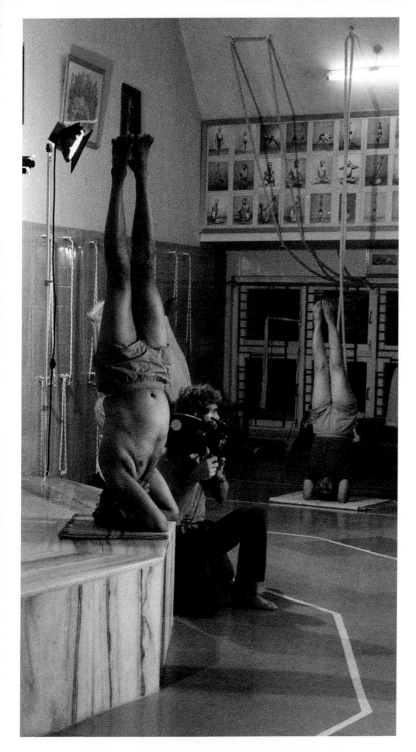

I remember they had this camp in Mahabaleshwar and there was this rock where Guruji said, "I want to do *Sirsasana* there." Everybody was like, oh my God, because there was a steep fall down. Not only did he do *Sirsasana*, but he did all the variations with a huge wind blowing. Those kind of challenges always came and as youngsters we were all game for it.

FAR

That was his courage and at the same time the confidence. It was not bravado, but I think it was that confidence going right up to the edge.

BM

When he used to take us to Mahabaleshwar it was a tremendous treat. Those were the days in the '60s and '70s. There were no props, only the wall and the rocks (at Mahabaleshwar). He would show us so many things that he would use. He would do yoga on the rocks. And it was tremendous to see that it was probably his way of doing yoga just as Patañjali looked at nature, and picked up poses from nature from the fish, from the animals, from the dog, from the tree.

FJP (Father Joe Pereira)

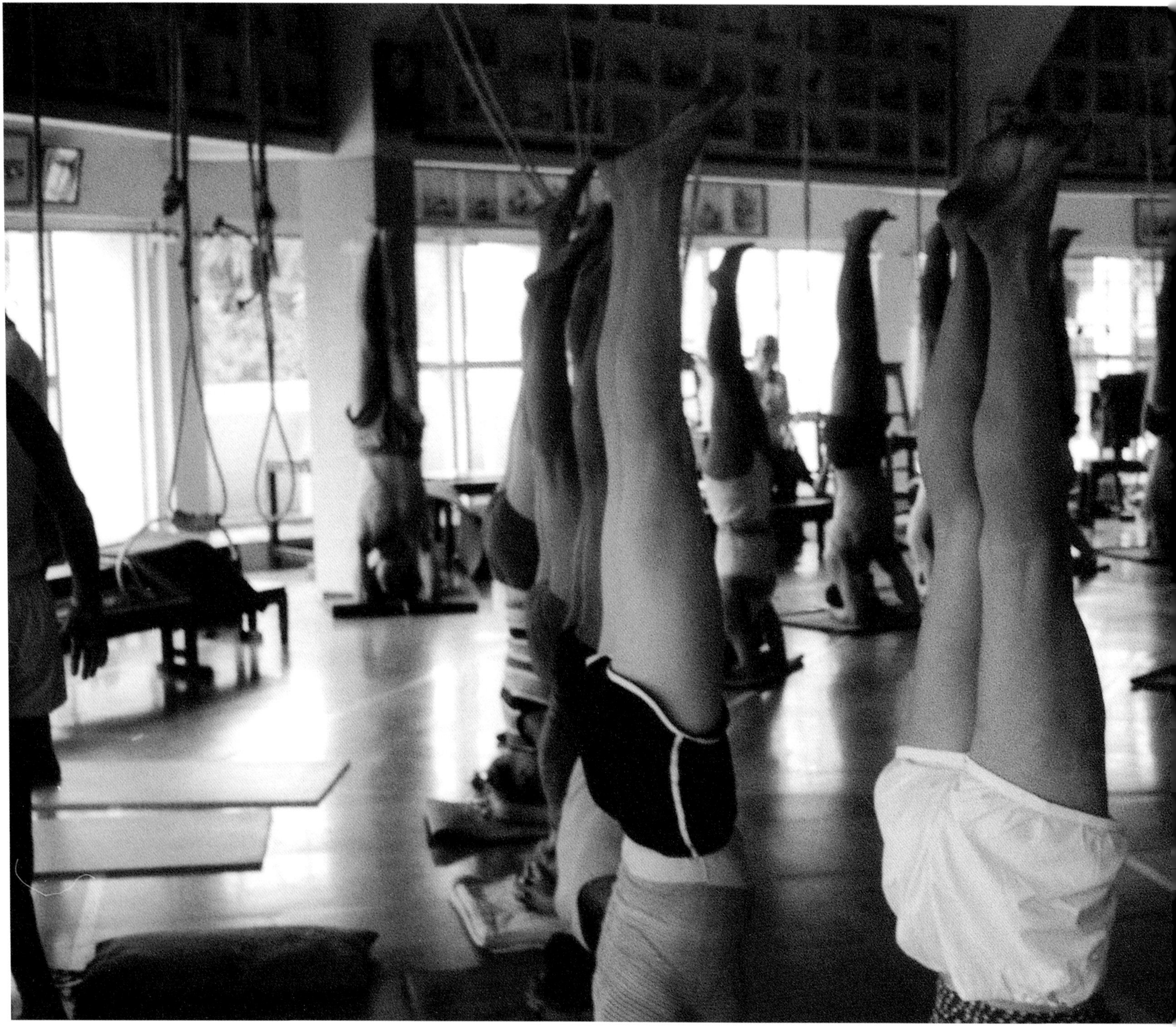

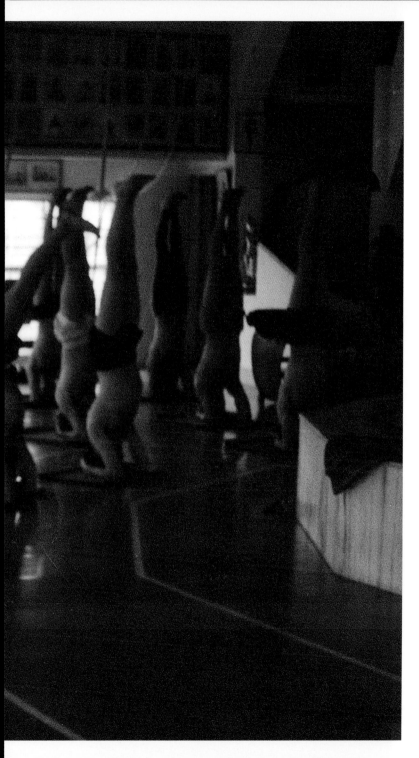

The first time I came to study with Guruji from Japan I understood very little English. I had only done 3 months of yoga in Japan and it was not Iyengar yoga. My friend and I had been taught to do *Sirsasana* balancing just on the edge of the forehead, so when we came to Pune we were doing head balance like this. As we didn't understand English, he didn't say anything to us, but with his leg he hit our backs so we fell over. This happened 3 days in a row. Finally we thought something must be wrong. My Japanese friend and I noticed that our eyes were red when we came down. Then we noticed that he was not taking anyone else out of *Sirsasana* and they were all on the crown of the head. None of them had red eyes. We also started doing like this. He didn't kick us out of head balance anymore and we had no more red eyes! He wanted us to learn by observing and doing.

NY (Naoko Yagyu)

He always had a twinkle in his eye in those days, no matter how fierce his behaviour. He pushed me over out of headstand, having told me earlier to come down if I lost his correction. I had been afraid to come down early in a class with Guruji. I fell sideways to the floor, more embarrassed and somewhat ashamed than anything else. He had made it clear that I had not done as he asked, and he always meant what he said.

PL

Mary Palmer had been host to the violinist Yehudi Menuhin in Ann Arbor in 1971. When the subject of yoga came up she mentioned to Menuhin that she was doing yoga and he asked her if she had *Light On Yoga* by BKS Iyengar. She said she did, but that it was way too difficult. He then said that if she was serious about yoga then she had to go study with him. She managed to get to Pune and was determined to find Guruji and take his classes. At that time he was teaching in the small courtyard at his house.

She appeared for the class but he said she could only watch. She went every day for three weeks and still was only allowed to watch. At the end of the third week he looked at her and said "I will put you in *Sirsasana* but if you come down before I say you can come down, then you will please go away and not come back again." Understand that Mary had never stayed in headstand longer than two or three minutes tops, but she was determined, so she stayed for 15 minutes and he then said she could come down. That was the beginning of a long and fruitful friendship.

JW

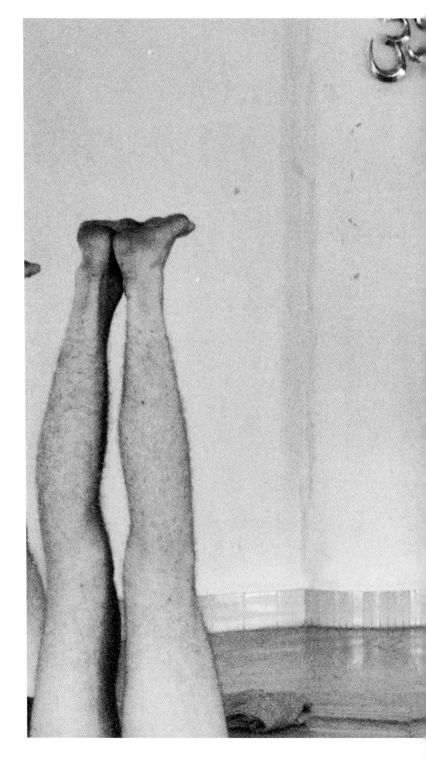

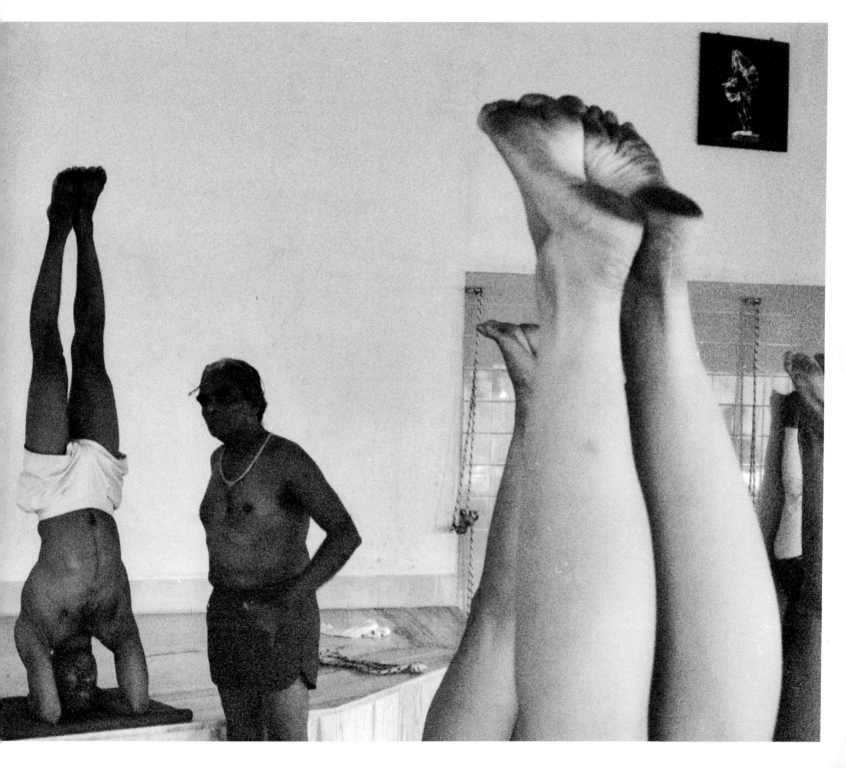

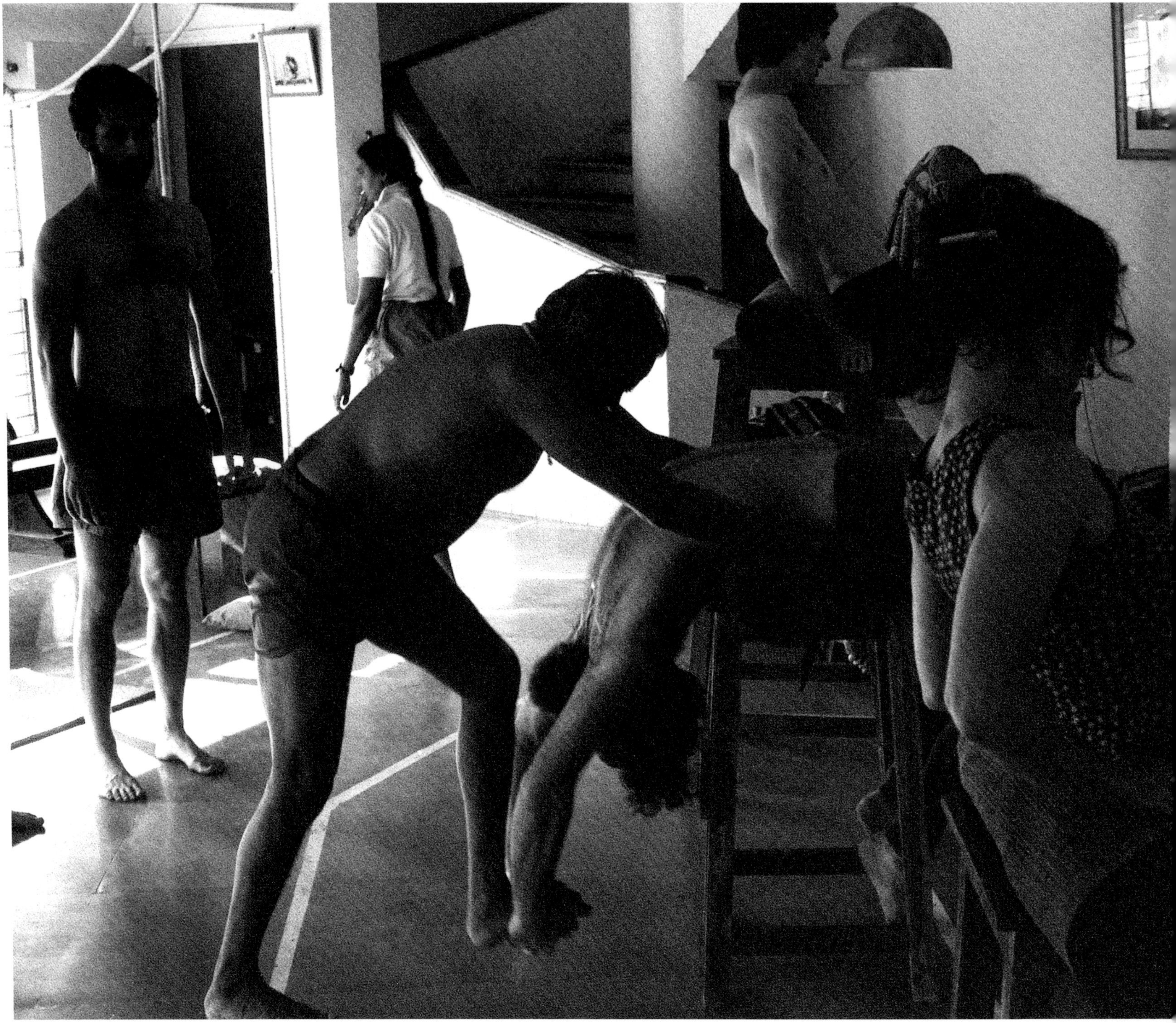

In the early days we did not have any props. He used to use his hands. He used to help and he had no props, no ropes, no belts. So backbends would be done using his hands for us to drop back instead of using the ropes that we use now. And he would pull us up. He would make us do the backbend 2, 3 or 4 times and then go to the next one, third one, fourth one, fifth one and so on and so forth. This would continue until the whole class had done it. Actually when he was teaching (before the Institute), everything was manipulated using his hands. Absolutely no props. I don't recall anything. It was all manipulated with his hands. And you never realised how well you did because he just knew what to do.

BM

Even when he was standing on those in *Supta Virasana*, most people didn't know how he placed the feet. Where to put pressure and where not to put the pressure, how much pressure is required. It is very, very interesting. People are looking and thinking he's shouting and hitting. Hitting was to the correct spot. Always the perfect spot. His eyes were very sharp. Oh! His eyes always knew exactly what was happening.

VD

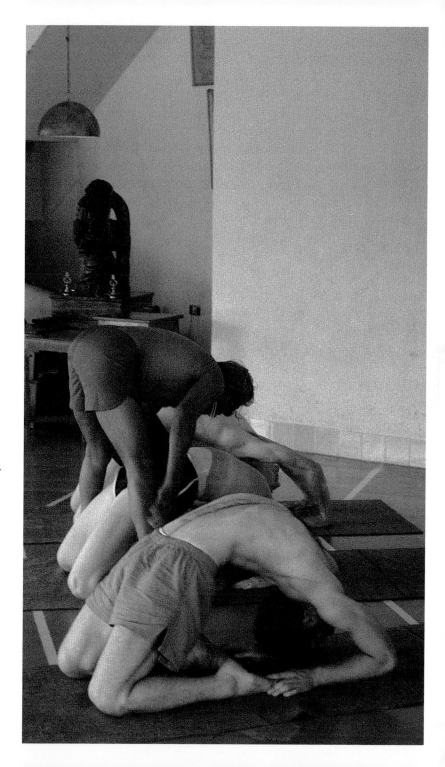

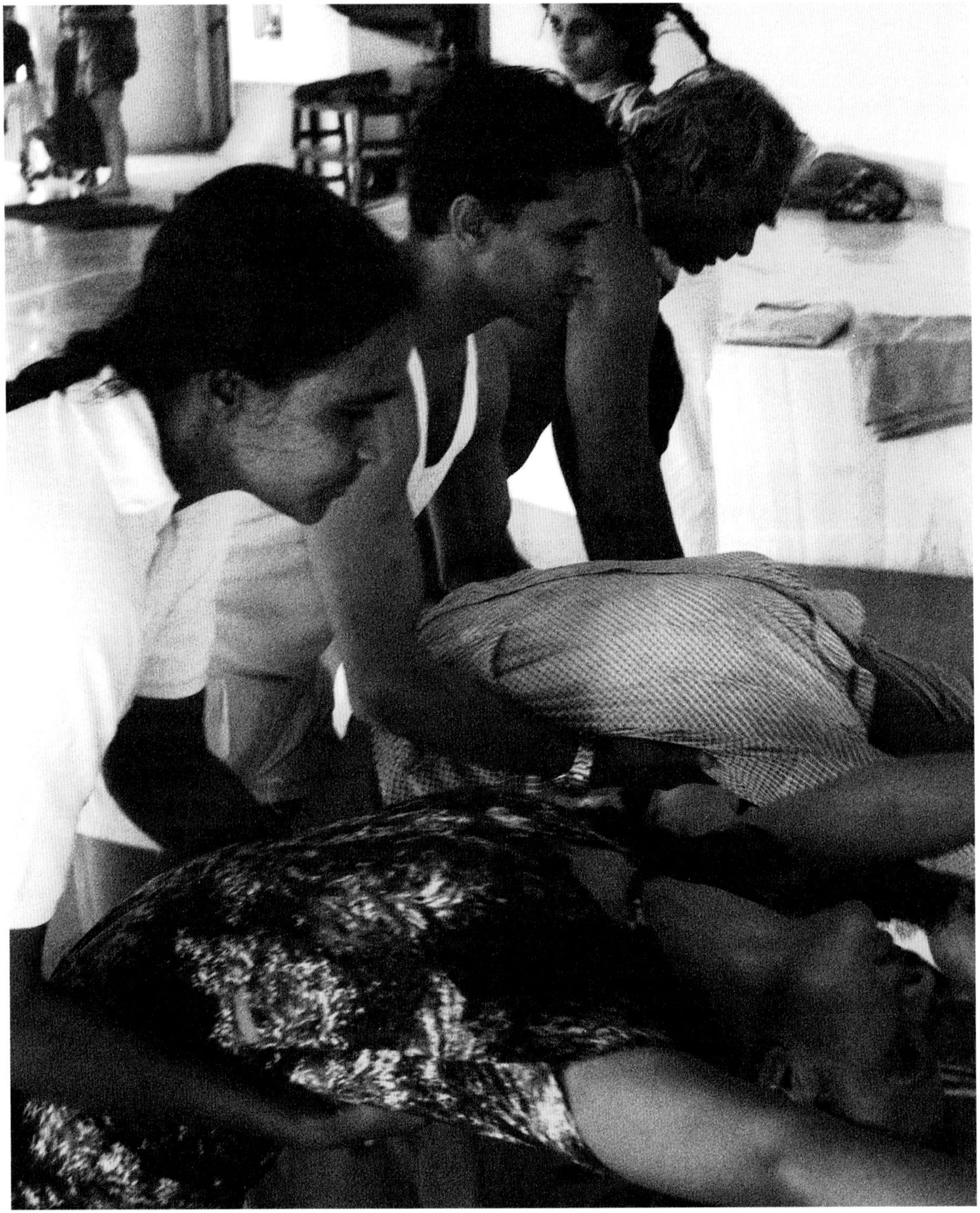

Guruji was very fast and efficient. In a group of 30 people he could adjust them all. That's when you knew the power of the man, the strength that he had. Even in a difficult twisting pose like *Ardha Matsyendrasana*, he would tie you up into knots or he would be lifting you up in full arm balance, or flipping you over to *Viparita Chakrasana* and he would do it very fast.

JB

He was unique so his classes were unique. His methodology, his way of teaching, his use of props, all were new and exciting. His way of doing yoga was nothing like the yoga I had experienced before his classes. He would go around and correct every student often and in every pose. He monitored us closely, he corrected us constantly and he kept us humble at all times. Nothing escaped his vision and, if he wanted to, he would turn that intensity and vision on you personally and you would learn how to work with yourself, and how to work with him. He really cared about us and if we stuck with him then he was always there for us. You always felt that he was talking directly to you even if he wasn't. He didn't let you slack off for a moment. He had an incredible amount of pure energy.

JW

On the face of it, this cache of black and white photos of when our Institute first opened, is simply a record of yoga classes in progress. Yet it has turned out to be an invaluable rare documentation of everything the world of yoga needs today—a zealous commitment to the student and to the subject, a deep knowledge of the student's body and mind. It's a visual record of guru-shishya parampara.

As yoga becomes more popular in these instantaneous times, especially as a method of wholistic healing, it is important that new generations realise that yoga is not a gross performance or routine drill, as can be seen in these captured moments of Guruji's subtle adjustments.

ZZ (Zubin Zarthoshtimanesh)

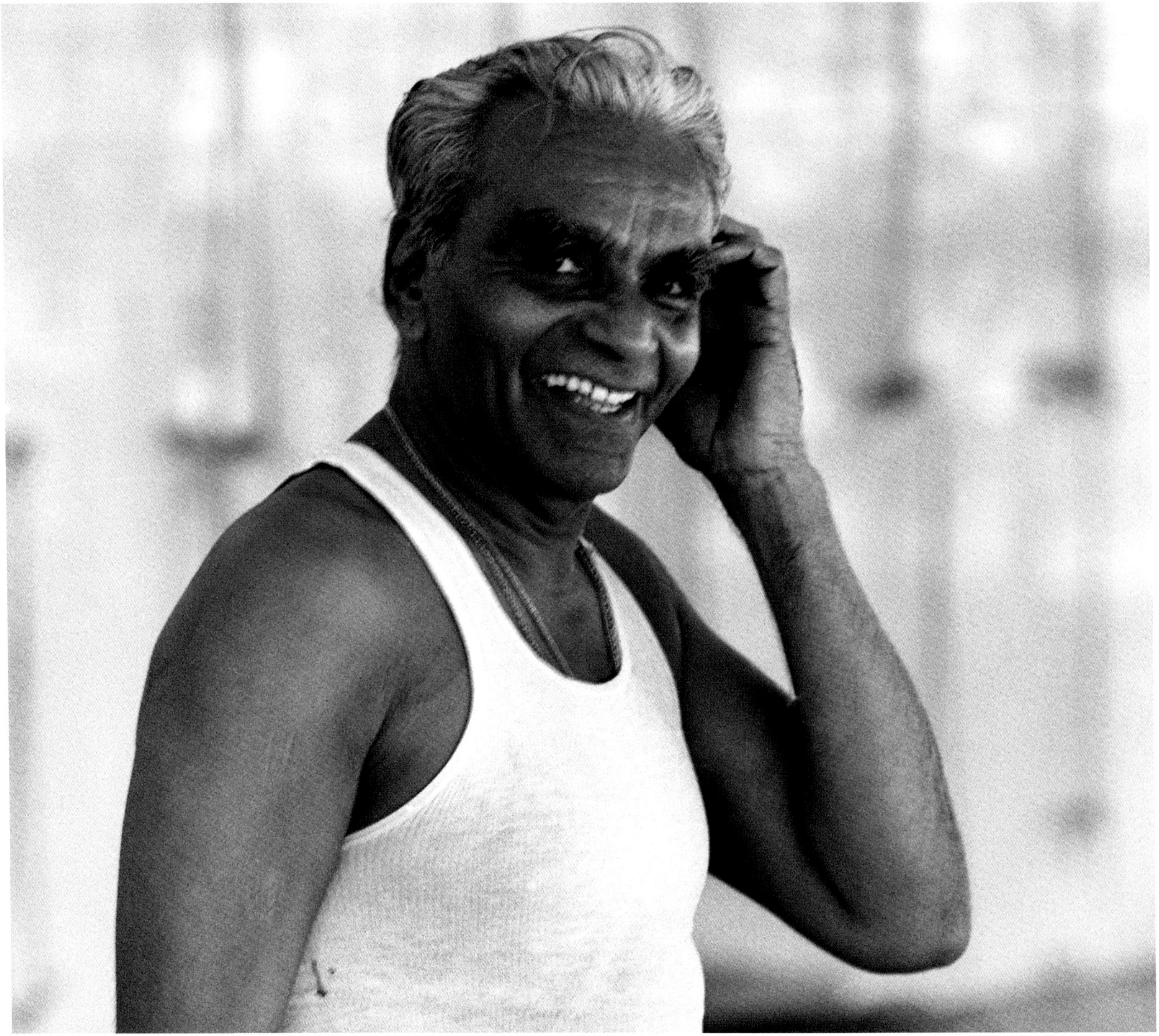

Sometimes we used to go on picnics with Guruji and his family. I was very surprised that a person like him would take the time to go with students for trips out of the city. There we had the chance to talk to him and he was compassionate and kind to everyone. Just as he could be strong and demanding in the class, he could be equally gentle and interested in everyone outside the class. The possibility of knowing this other side of Guruji helped me to have more respect and affection for him.

GG

I had the good fortune of hosting Guruji at my house. Guruji was such a non-demanding person as a guest. Of course, for me, he was like my father and I wanted to give the best. When he stayed with us, he was just a part of the family sitting comfortably, cracking jokes with the children, making me feel at ease by just saying "I feel at home here!" It was like he was an honoured guest but a part of the family who you are so happy to have! He'd try all the dishes because he knew I had made them. His simplicity was unique as I cannot imagine anyone as great as him being so much at ease and completely unpretentious.

ND (Neeta Datta)

In class I was almost petrified but then after class he transformed into this wonderful man with this beaming smile who could enjoy going out for a party or enjoy a slab of chocolate or enjoy eating ice cream and inducing us to eat as well and slapping you on the back and smiling. It was basically him that pushed me on.

FAR

The first time I was at RIMYI I told him I was attending a Yoga conference in India that he was teaching at. He said, "Good, come with me and two Indian ladies in the taxi." From the moment we were in the taxi it was like there was a radical transformation from stern yoga master to the most engagingly brilliant and funny person any of us could ever hope to meet. I had a good supply of stories and I remember well his turning around in the front seat to join us in our laughter. At the conference at first most people were afraid of him and wouldn't sit at the table with him in the dining room. By the end of the week it was the opposite. You had to run to get a seat there as all wanted to be with him. The same thing happened in his classes, only faster. Naturally it only took one day for his classes to be packed.

JP

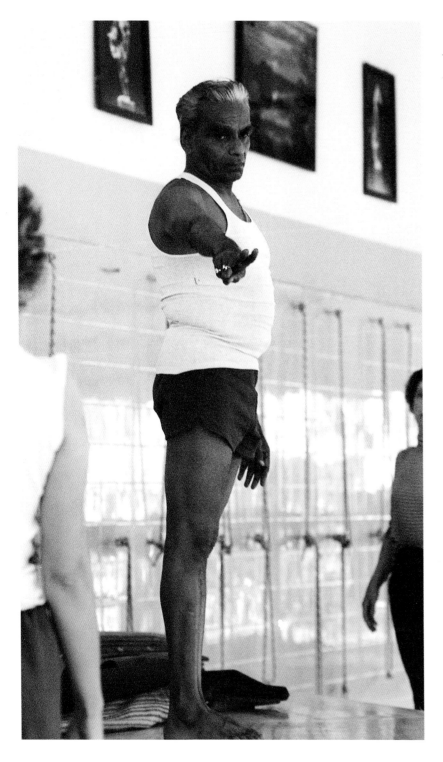

Yes, everyone was afraid of Guruji in the early days, including myself. We were afraid of him, but for me, I got used to him very soon. This was because as a child, my parents were strict. We are an orthodox Parsi family, so my parents were strict. I was brought up in a convent school and my teachers were strict. They were nuns, so you had to do your hair this way—no clips, no fashion, no short dresses. So it was a strict atmosphere at home and at school, and if I got a strict guru it was nothing new to me. In the classes, if you deserved a slap, you deserved a slap. But we accepted it. We knew it was a part of the training so we accepted him completely. It was not new to me and I did not ever feel offended. I used to get surprised when foreigners used to start crying when Guruji would hit them or shout at them they would start crying. I used to get very surprised. Hasn't their mother or father ever scolded them? He is just like a father to you. And if he scolds you it's not something new. In fact, it's for your own good... and psychologically I think we are very normal.

CD (Colle Dastur)

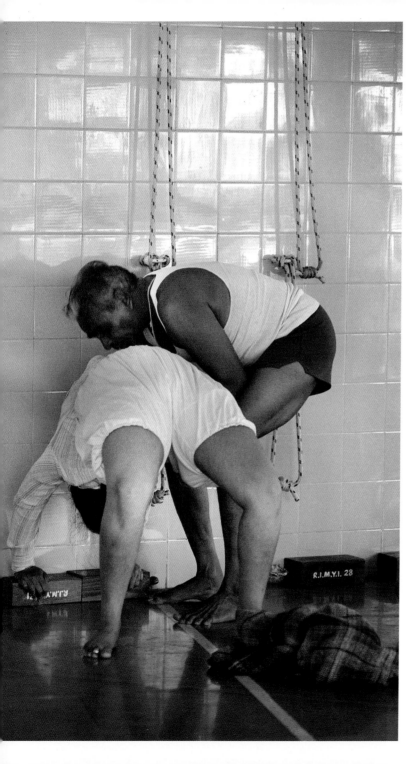

I was always aware that he was watching. I will give you one example. I was in the medical class with Guruji and Geeta. I had a pupil and I thought this pupil is doing very well, I'm glad. I was thinking this to myself when a big bang came onto my back just then at that moment that I was feeling proud of this student I was teaching. Then he was telling me, "40 years you are with me, and you don't know how to teach!" That means the ego came down then. I said, "Guruji, it's been 50 years." He said, "50 years?" I said, "Yes Guruji, 50 years with you and I was only 20 years with my father!" And he started laughing. He never allowed our egos to get inflated. He brought us down to earth, he was very practical, and today I remember him very often.

CD

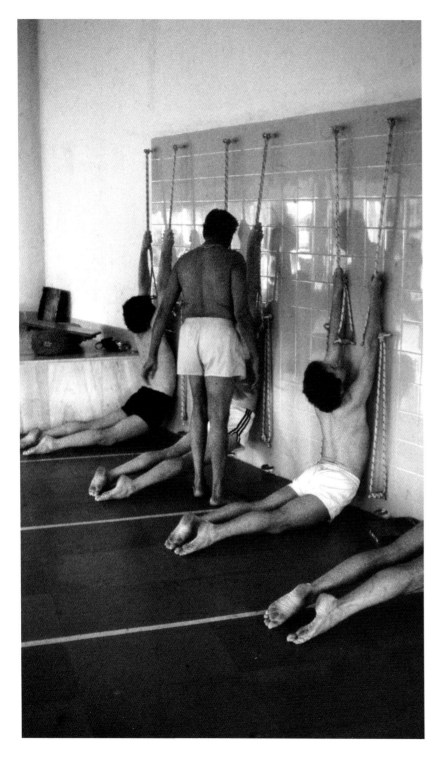

Guruji called the rope work the Celestial Poses. They allow you the closest opportunity to experience the principle of *akasha*, just space. You are in free fall, in space and saved, there is a line to save you, a safety clause of sorts. I can remember him saying that if your backbend practice recedes, regain the practice first using ropes. They don't harm, they add space into the body, into the spine, into the mind.

Children innately see the great purpose of ropes, as soon as they enter the hall they run to them, they swing, they play. They never need to be shown how.

The ropes are also a situation of intelligently applied brakes and restraints, giving form to pure space. You give yourself free fall and then modify that free fall by applying the ropes in different degrees of restraint. The ropes can be the safety harness of a mountain climber, they can also be used as manacles, shackles, you can apply a rope so it binds you to a wall, and then go with gravity, the release, the extension, the freedom then is very localised and specific.

SQ (Stephanie Quirk)

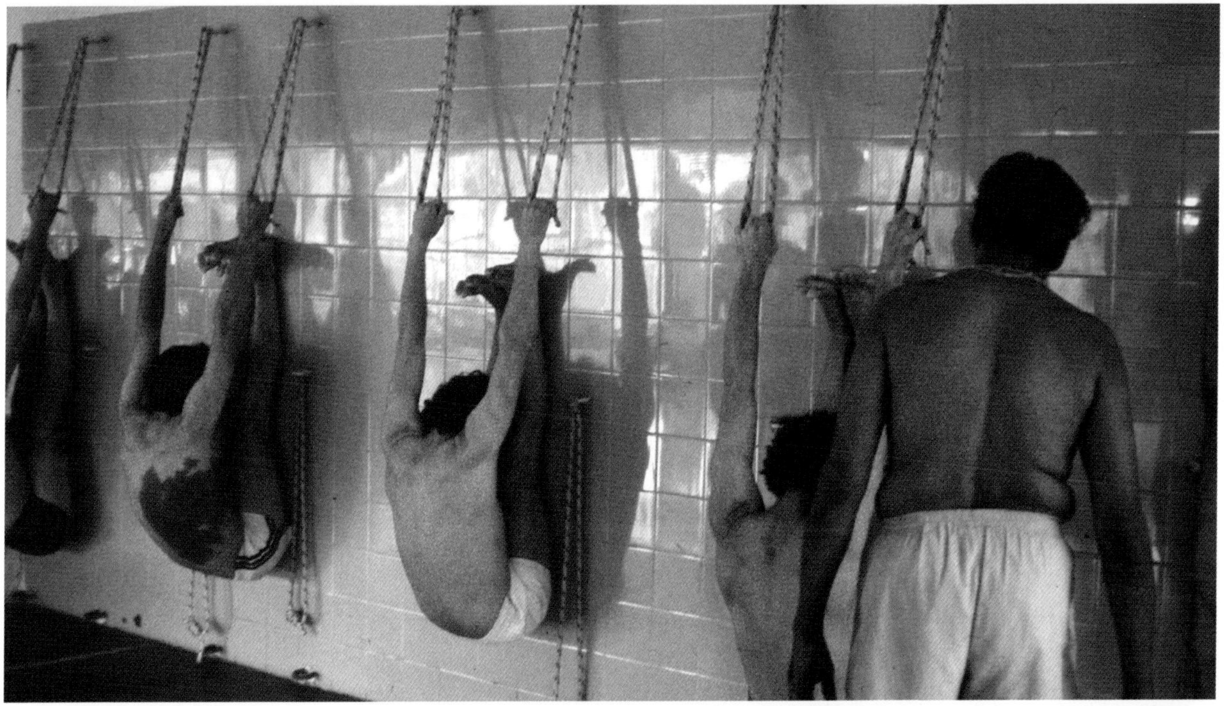

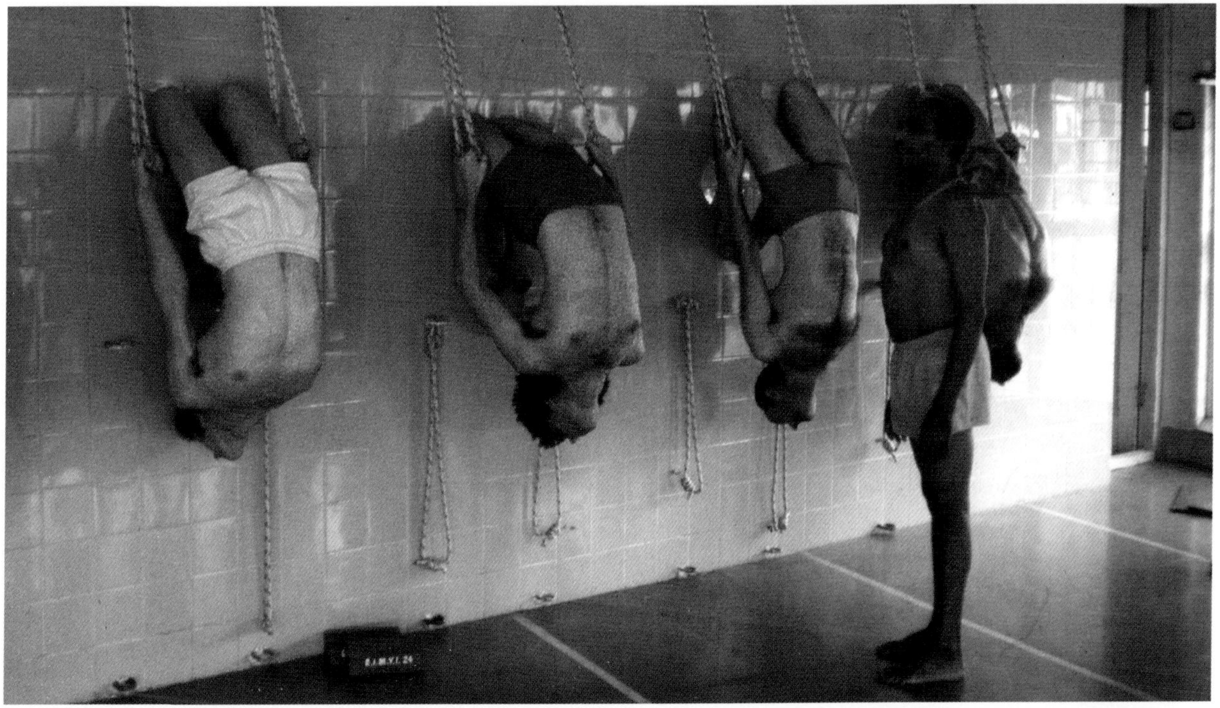

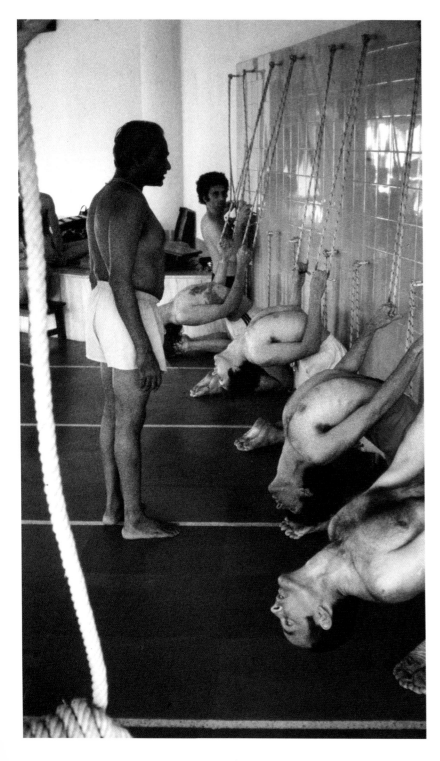

Rope *asanas* are quite often used to create preparatory actions and movements in poses. Standing poses practised with the ropes teach us to refine and correct our balance and focus.

Most notably, the ropes teach us depth in backbends, where the ropes train us to move into unknown areas of our body and mind. The ropes train us to undo what Geeta Iyengar calls the "inner knots" of the body and the mind. The ropes teach us to move beyond the horizons of bondage that attach us to fixed states of consciousness into new perspectives and spheres of understanding.

PS (Peter Scott)

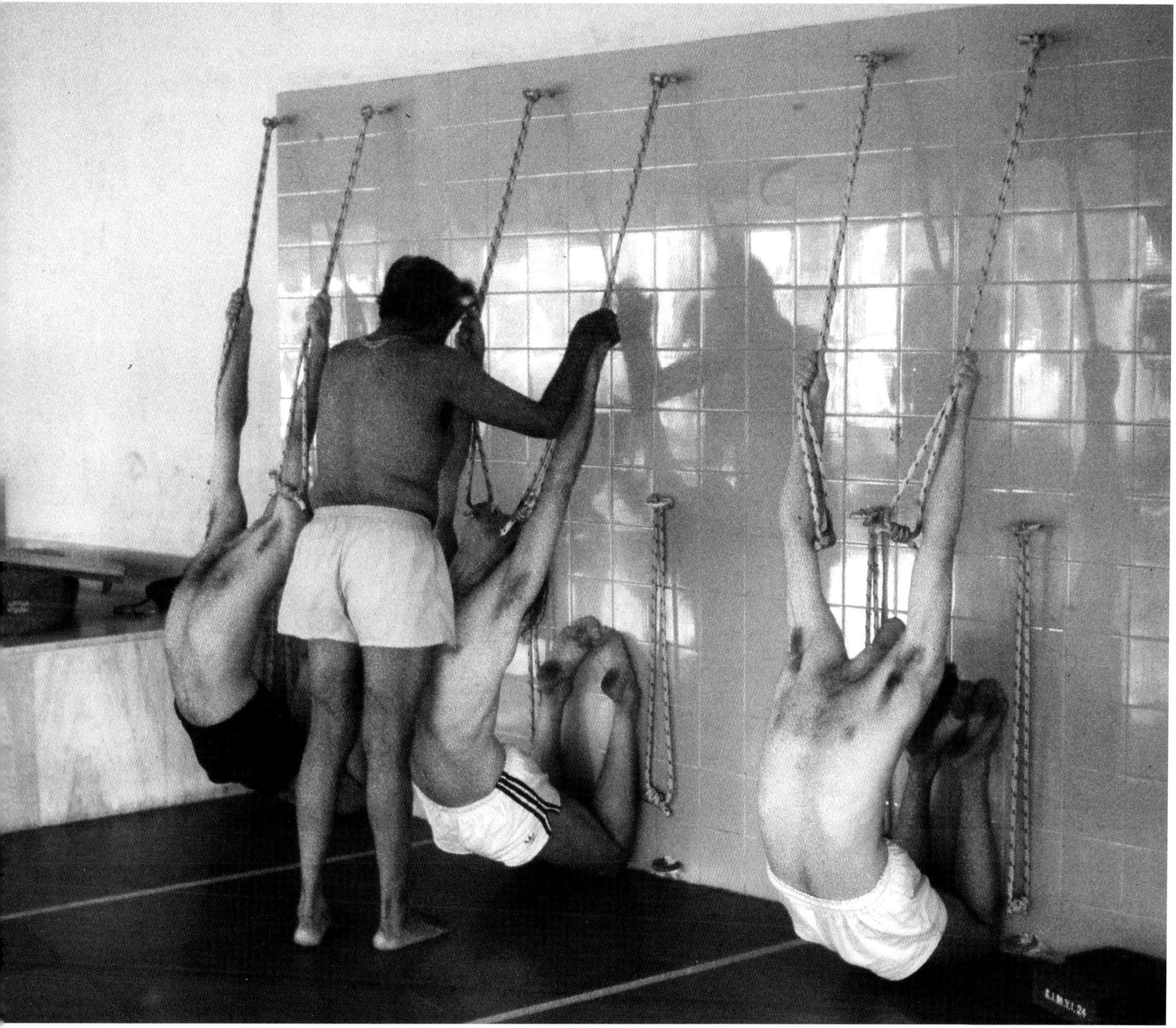

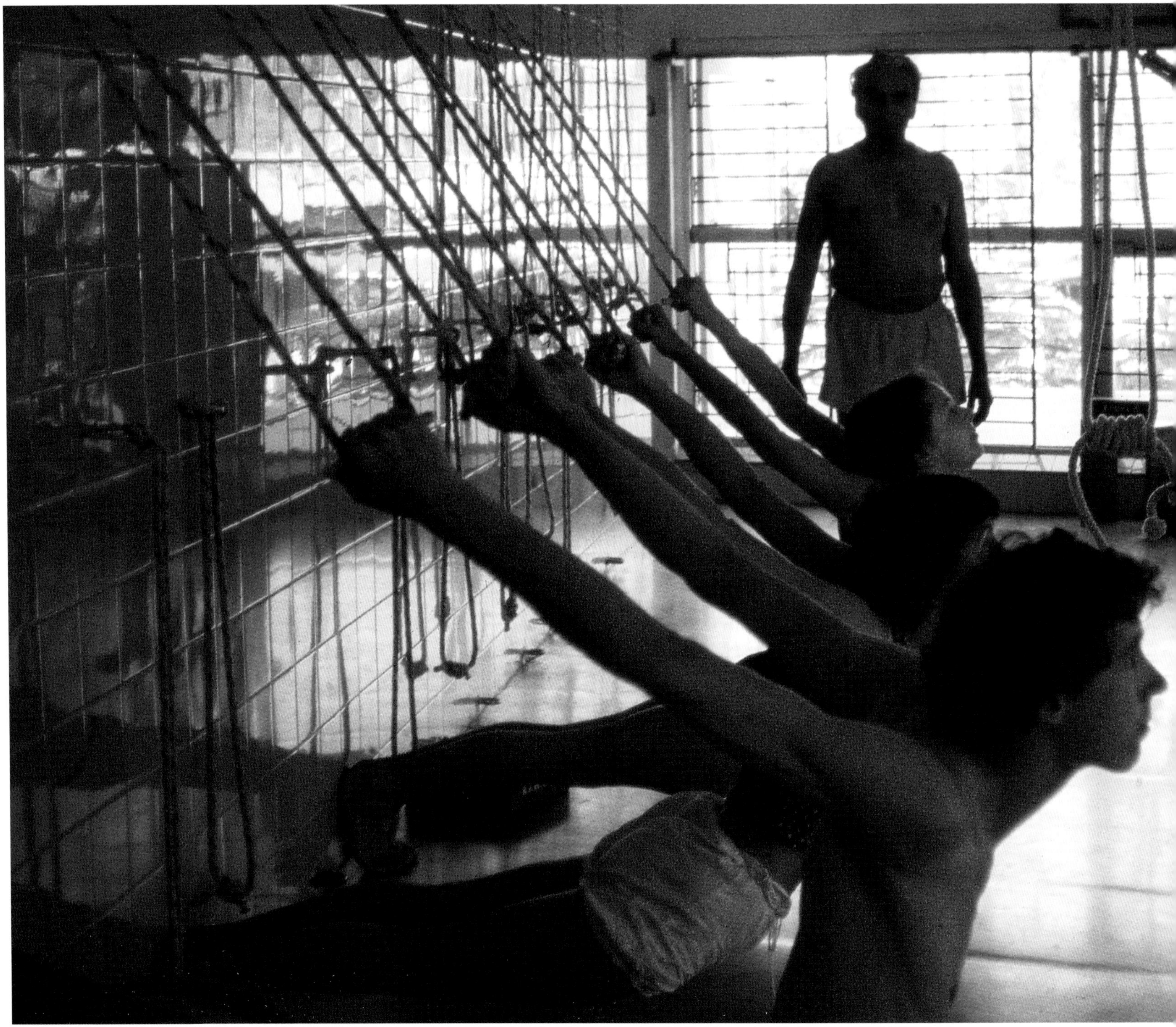

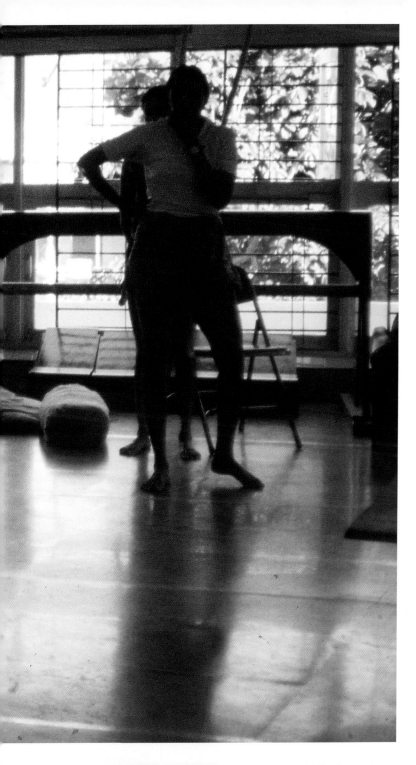

We would be hanging off the wall ropes in Rope 1, as in this photo. Our heels were against the wall, with our bodies curving away from the wall from our heels through our tailbones and pelvis, then arching back through the middle trunk, chest and head toward the wall. Guruji would admonish us, "Tailbone in, chest up!" We tried, but not satisfied with our efforts, Guruji would then walk down the line between the wall and us. He stopped behind each student and rolled our upper arms in before taking hold of our hands, which in turn held the ropes. With the ball of his foot he gave two or three pushes to each of our sacrums to get the measure of each student's mobility. We gently bounced with the movement of his foot. The final push was stronger and sharper, and tailbones moved in.

If we were lucky, there might be an additional push in the center of the dorsal spine. Chests opened followed by relieved out-breaths.

BC

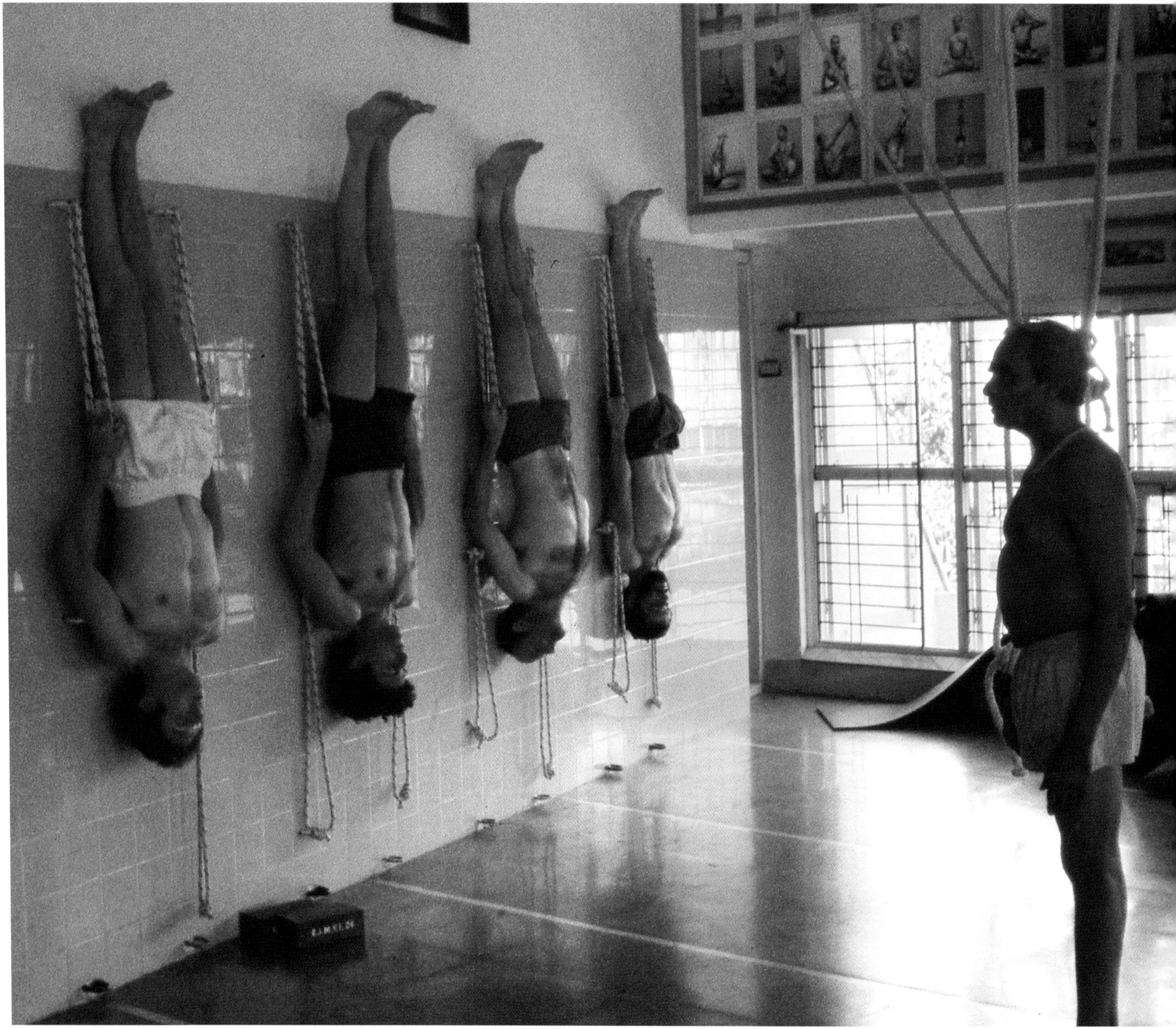

The wall ropes were used quite a lot in the early days. We often used the ropes to prepare for the classes as the effect of the pose using the ropes was much enhanced. As the class size was much smaller, it was easier for Guruji to have us do many new variations of the poses using the ropes. You never knew what he was going to teach in the class. For us it was all new. There were so many variations of backbends, forward bends and inversions.

I remember clearly the first time we did the rope *Sirsasana* like in the photo on the left. A friend of mine was rather fearful of doing the pose. Geeta came over with a helping hand and admonished her, "Get over your fear complex!" She had her repeat it several times and indeed she did get over it and actually came to like it—on rare occasions.

There was always a strong feeling of anticipation and eagerness before the classes. We loved them. Many of us planned our lives around how to be able to come back the next time!

JP

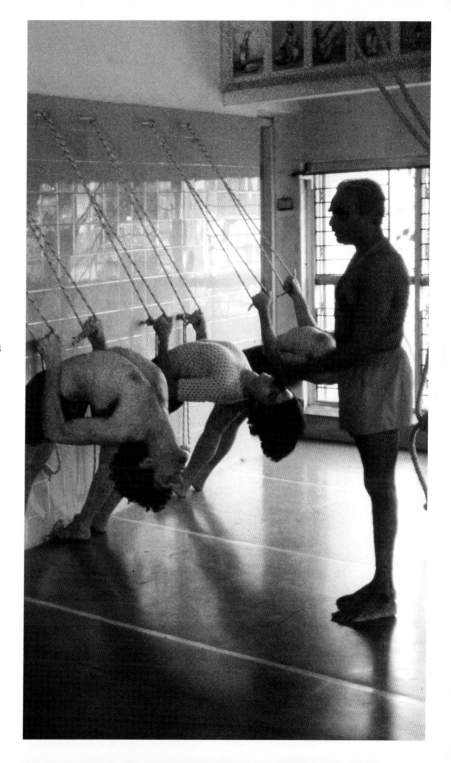

In the '70s at the Institute we sometimes were allowed to place our tape recorders on the stage to record the class. After Guruji died, I listened to some of those old recordings. I had almost forgotten the immense power and electrifying energy of his every word. There was no question about it—everyone gave their all in those classes.

JP

Guruji himself gave me the courage to teach, with the caveat to remain humble and to first practice myself what I was going to teach. He said to take other people's problems into my own body and learn from that, which I spent years doing. He encouraged us to experiment on ourselves, not on others and I still follow that advice. I was always in awe of his abilities, his discipline, his lightning fast corrections and his high standards for himself as a Yogi.

JW

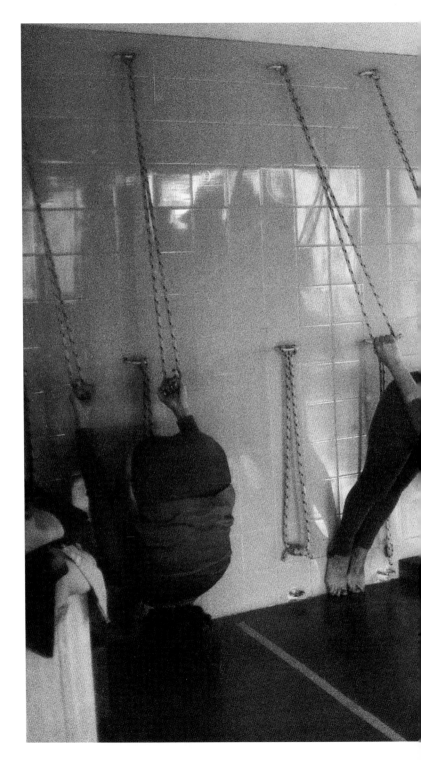

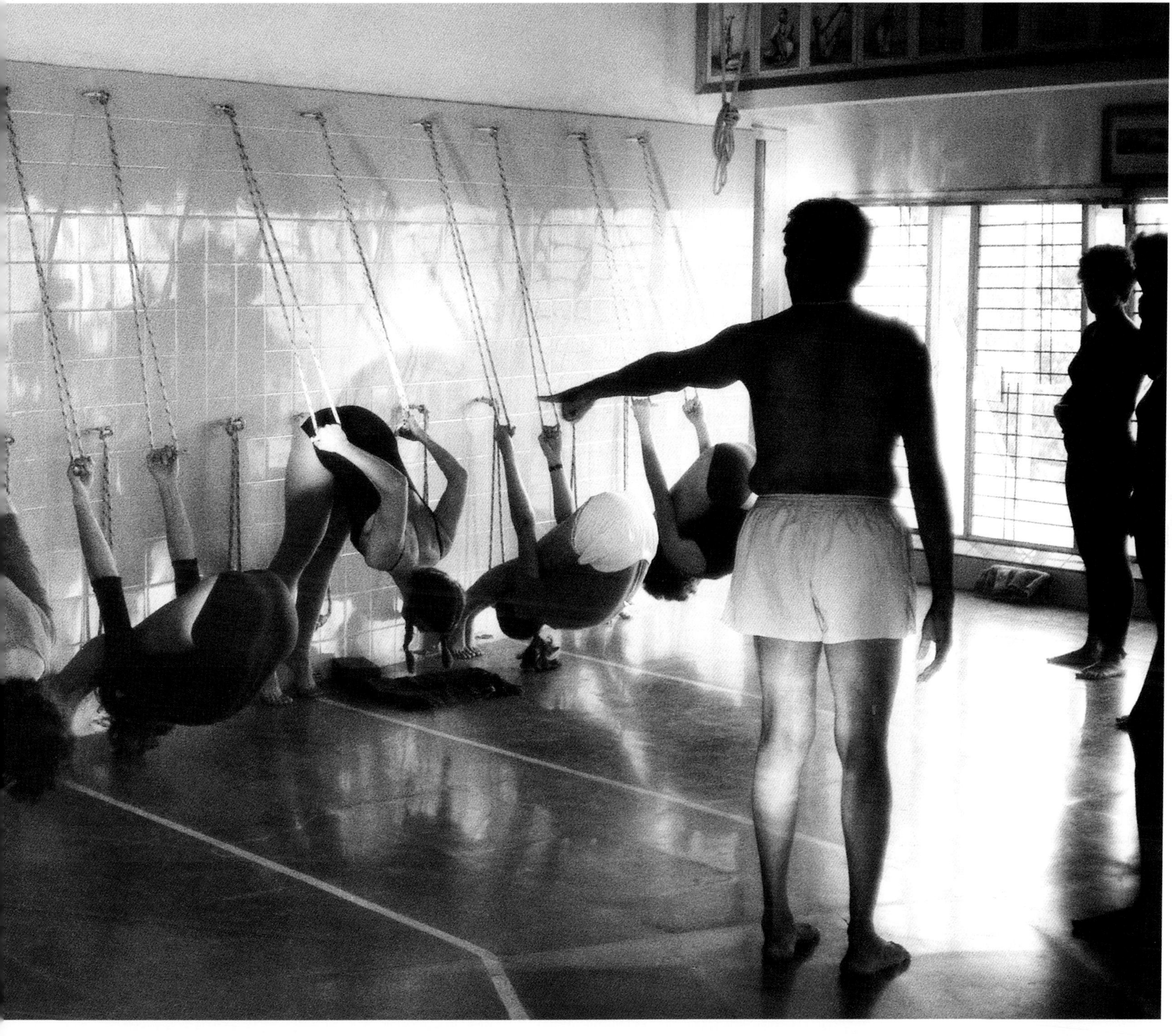

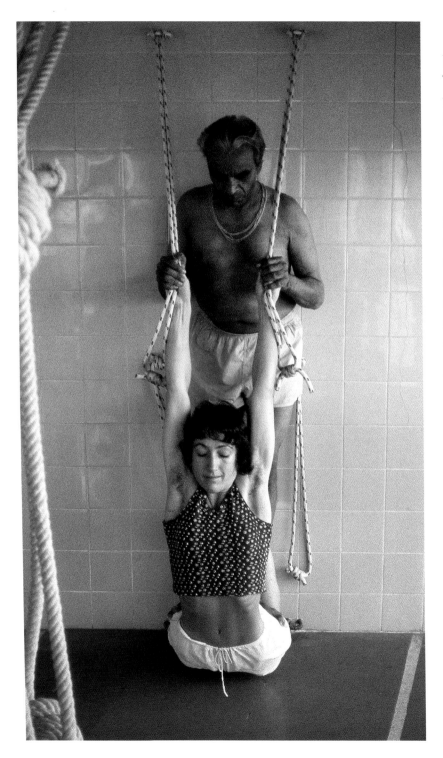

His classes were unique. Every class was a new discovery. There was always the excitement of discovering and understanding something new. He was never repetitive. Every time I thought I understood something, he had the ability to surprise us with something new.

GG

Back in the early days at my first intensive, Guruji was very feisty and intense! Yet what was always so amazing was his sense of humour and he was very kind and encouraging. He always knew the potential of the student and got them to do their utmost best. Most of the time, the students themselves never knew their capacity and would be amazed at their progress.

ND

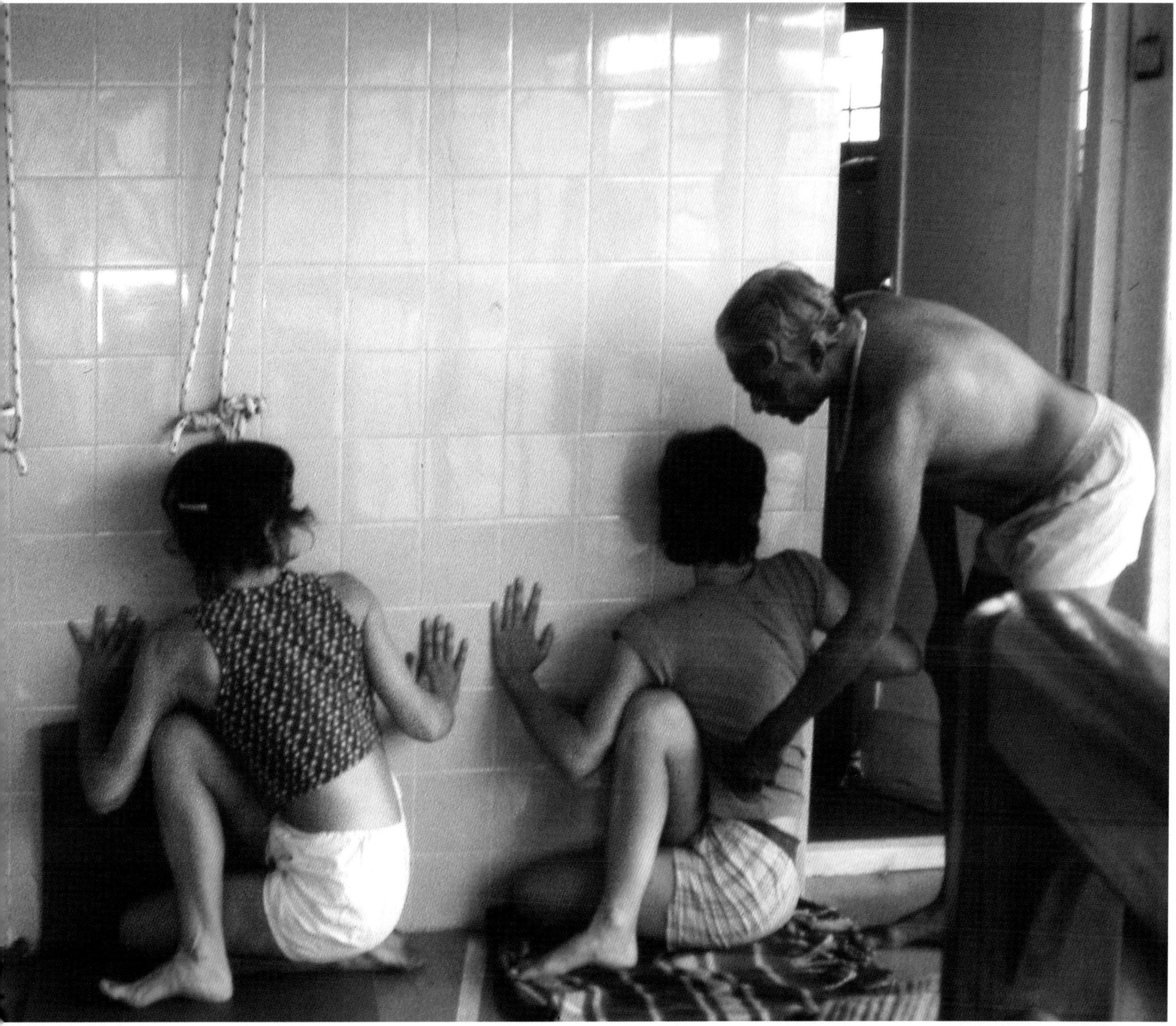

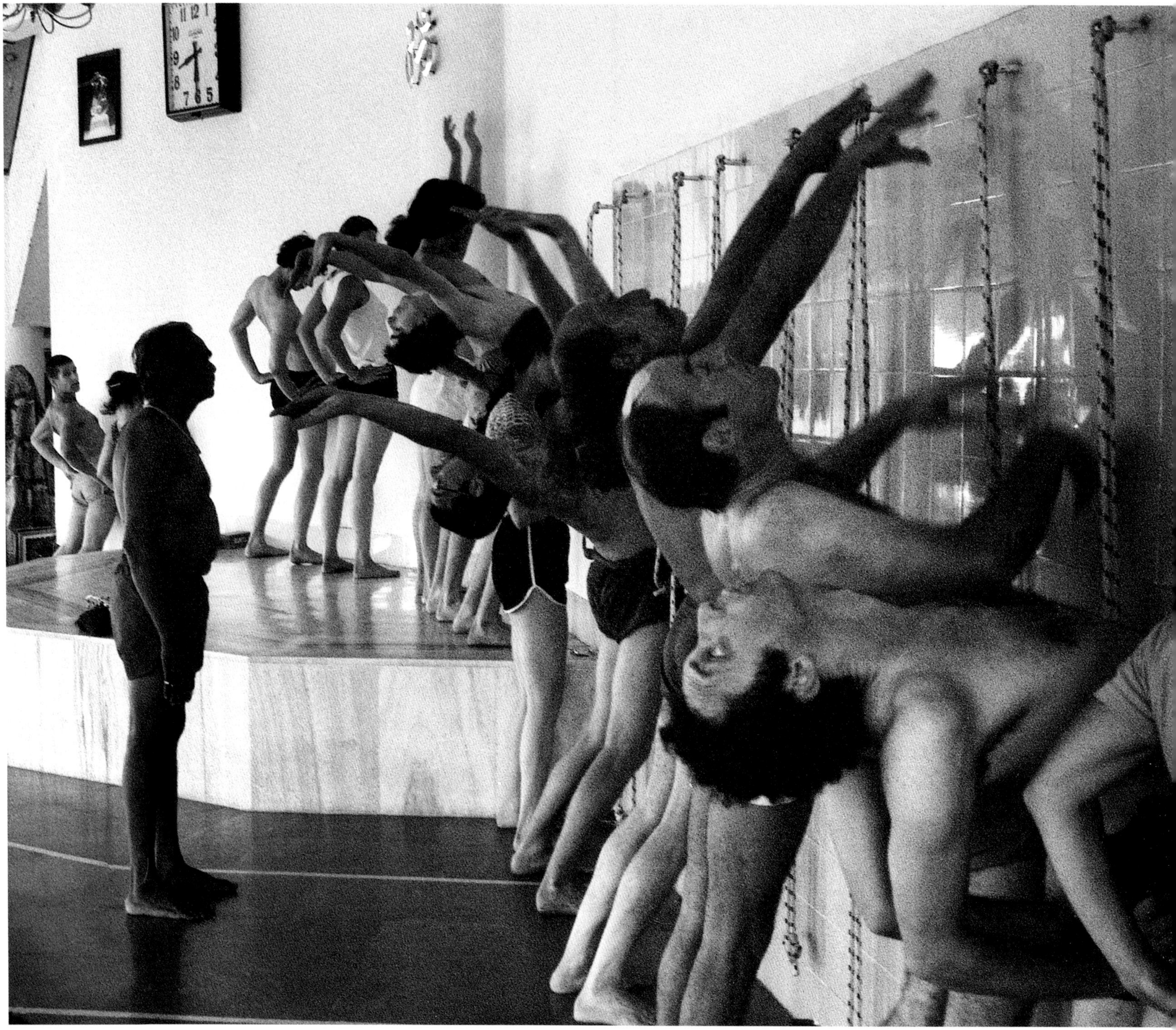

Guruji would stand in front of a student and look them in the eye and tell them what to do. He was intensely intense. He was fierce, he laughed, and we all felt seen by him. To be in the presence of someone who loved what they did and was able to maintain a presence of mind throughout the whole class was electrifying. It was a first. We never had the experience of being in the presence of someone like Guruji. He said what was on his mind, he wasn't trying to please people.

I completely trusted him. He was clearly my teacher. My devotion to him and to the Iyengar method deepened and matured. My devotion deepened, my practice deepened; it was a transformation really. I was transformed by his teaching and by my own practice.

PW

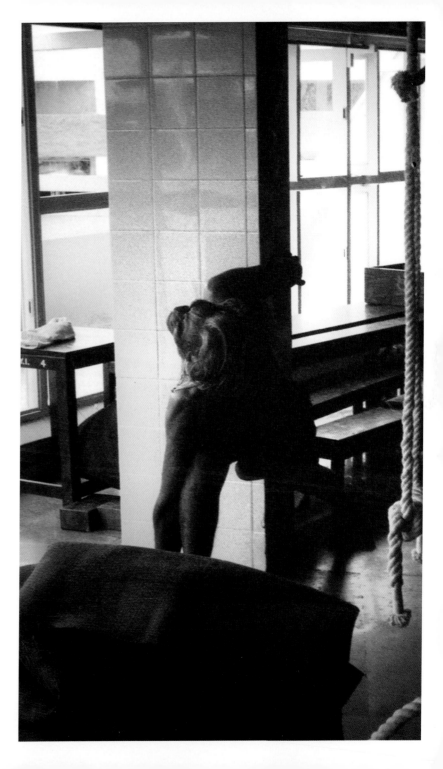

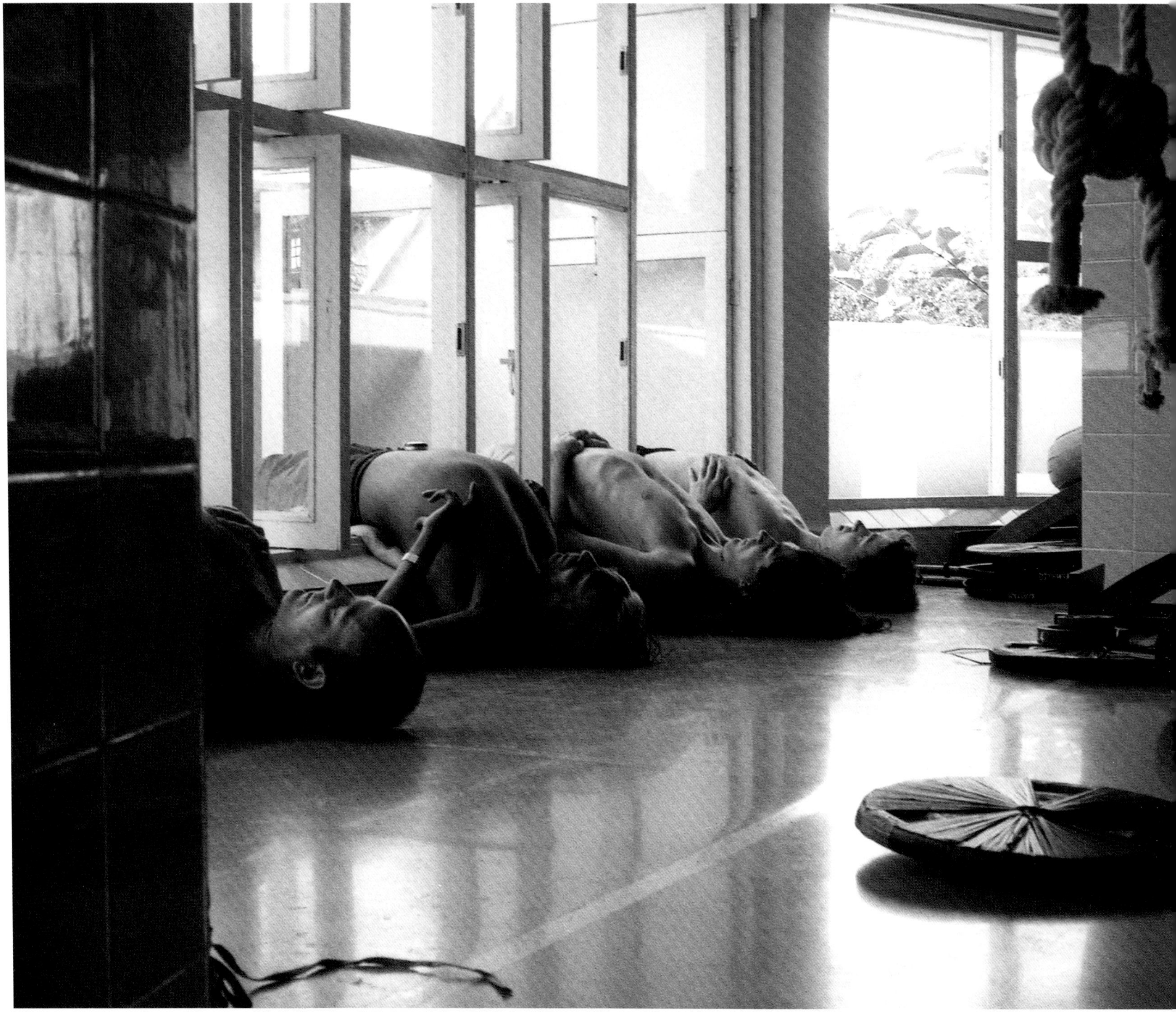

After a class while we were in *Savasana* he said, "Feel the coolness in the brain. See how the mind has gone inwards without any *mantra*, any meditation technique. Then slowly open the eyes and see how the mind is still inward, though the eyes are open."

A few of us were practising in the hall in the 70's one day when we saw Guruji finish his practice and go into *Savasana*. His body was perfectly aligned and completely at ease. However, after some time we were almost getting concerned as his breathing was undetectable and he was totally still. There was not even a flicker of an eyelid. There was absolutely no trace of movement. He looked so serene and internalised we did not want to disturb him. He was far away from us. And sure enough after an hour he quietly got up and walked away. He has said *Savasana* is the most difficult of them all.

JP

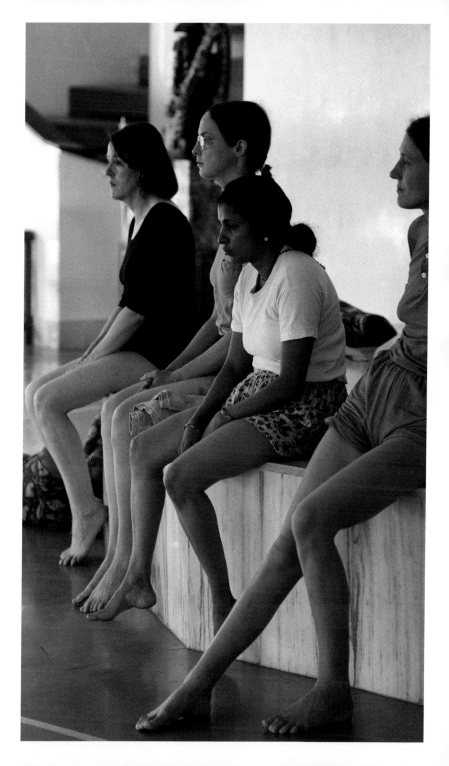

Guruji was so subtle and swift that it was very difficult for me to understand what he was saying in my early days. For example, if he said move the skin in this direction— it was a language that I did not understand. How can the skin move? After many years, I understood this instruction and the range of effects as well as penetration that it gave. Suddenly, what he expressed as space, ether seemed alive. The depth of his knowledge, experience, wisdom, his articulation, his touch gave him the ability to transfer his knowledge and experience to others. It was so fundamental in his teaching that we did not realise his work in the future might seem that like of a miraculous magician to those that never met him.

RM

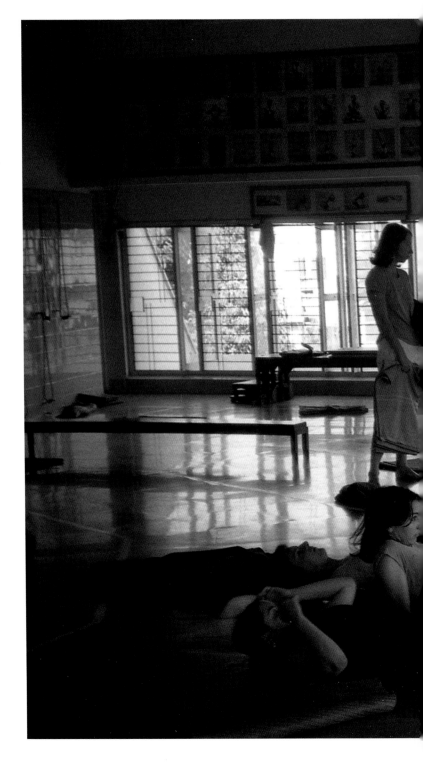

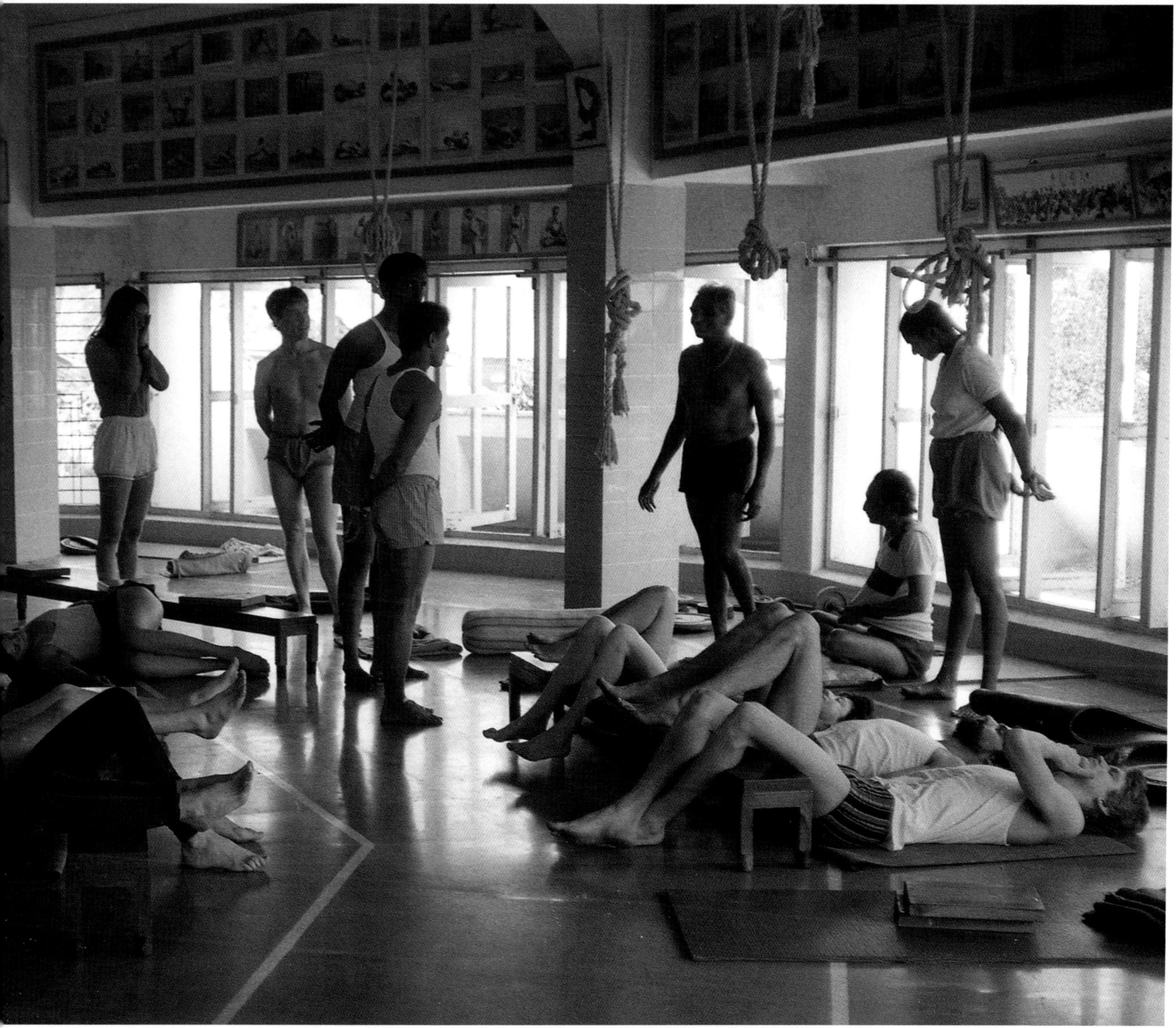

Guruji's Practice

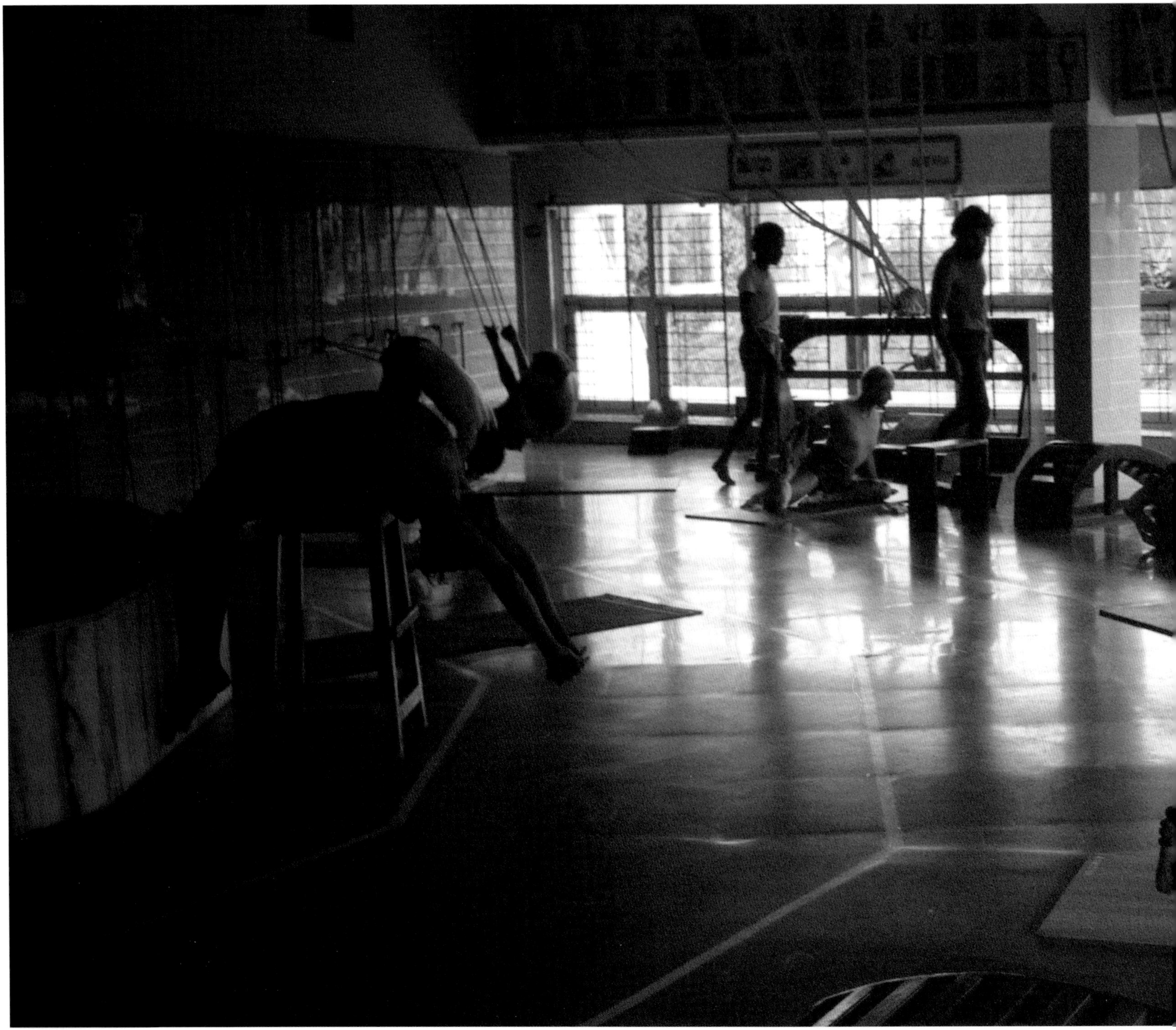

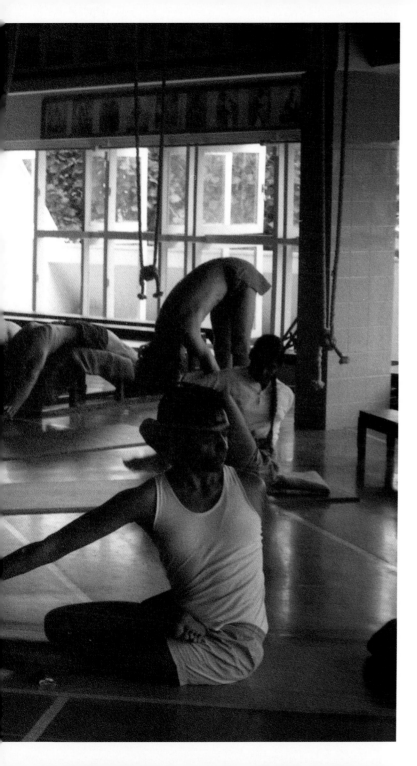

On Friday morning there would be no class and Guruji would be practising and we would practise with him. I mean with him, as in we were in the same hall. I do know that I was very excited on Fridays because I would think today he's going to do his backbends. Friday was his backbend day so to say. Once I saw him do 108 *Viparita Chakrasanas*, standing on the same spot. I got tired of counting, but he went on and on and on.

One of the attractions of that practice was also to keep looking at what he was doing. We did learn a lot, because then we would try to use the prop the way we saw him doing. And he would sometimes look from the corners of his eyes and see what we are doing. Sometimes he would call out and say, "Hey—that's not how you should be doing it. You should do it like this." There were not too many interruptions in his practice in those days. In later years he set out to teach more and more, he would be teaching Raya or Abhijata. It wasn't that kind of a teaching for us, but sometimes he would say something. Sometimes he would call us and say, "When I am doing this, do you know what I am experiencing? Do you know what is happening?" Then he would go on to explain how he was stretching, where the stretch would come. I think we didn't understand a lot of things. We tried to understand.

FAR

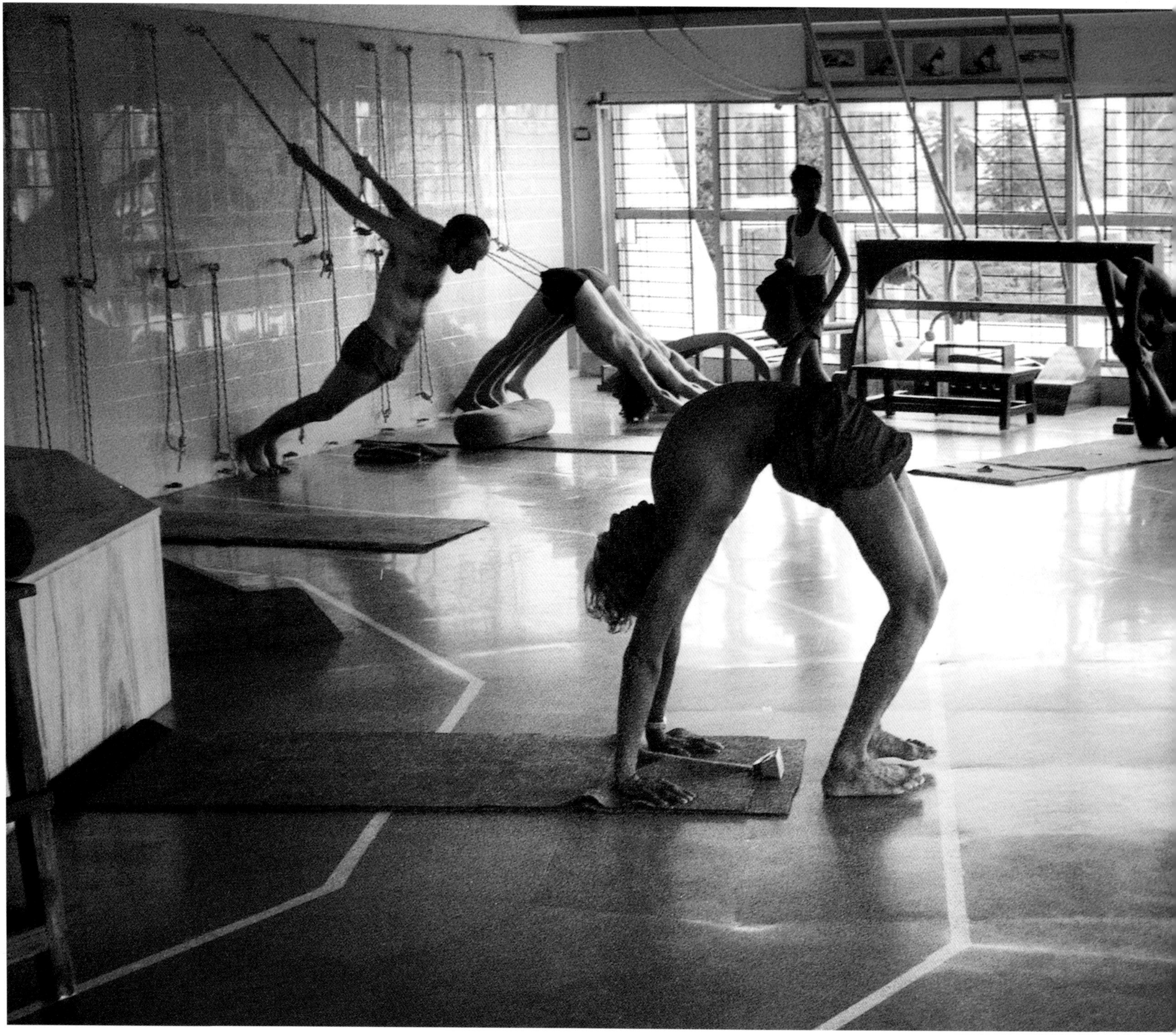

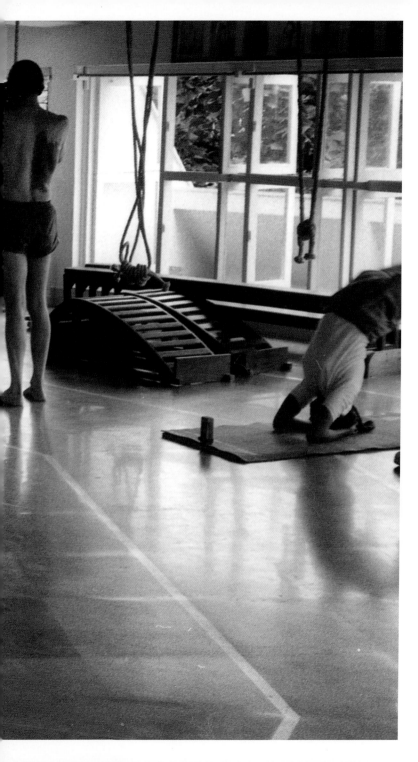

Sometimes when in the hall during the morning practice times, I would look across and see Guruji, he was in his own practice, not teaching anyone, not talking to anyone. A very strong thought would arise in my mind, "Who is that man?" Or really, where is he now. We all know, have experienced the communication, the teaching, the guidance that was Guruji. We all practise what he broadcasted, implored, guided, chided us to do, but sometimes I would catch sight of him alone just practising, "Where are you?" I always had a very strong sense that in his practice, he had his own private conversation. We only ever know what he wanted us to know about practice, but I began to see that that was not necessarily his own personal search, he has his own private conversation. He was in a constant, private dialogue, which really we know nothing of. It was a contrast as a lot of the time he seemed very present with us. There wasn't ever anything held back about him, he was totally present and very, very generous with his time—yet, alone he went silently on with his practice. Where are you, *gate gate paragate* (...gone to the other shore.)

SQ

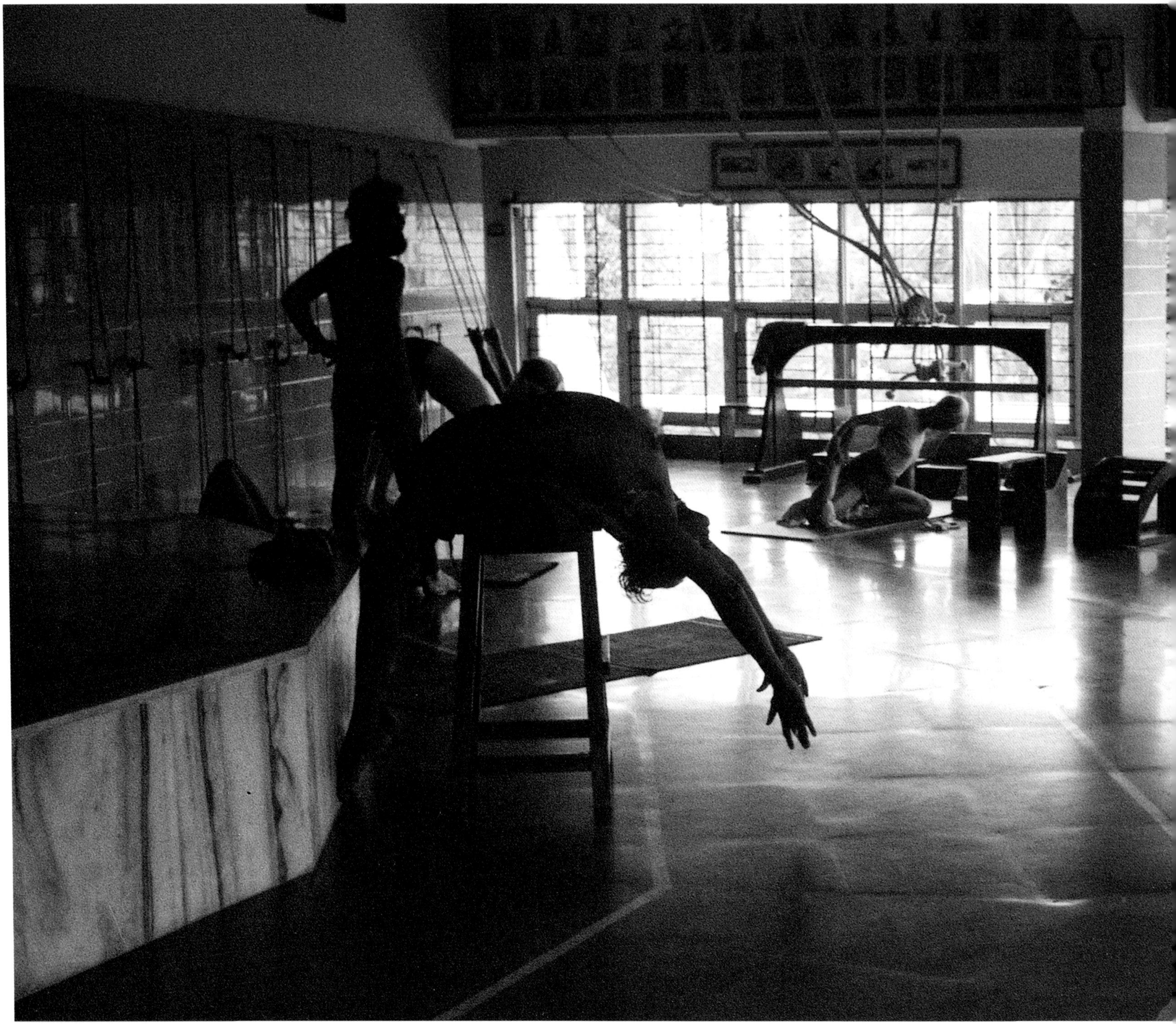

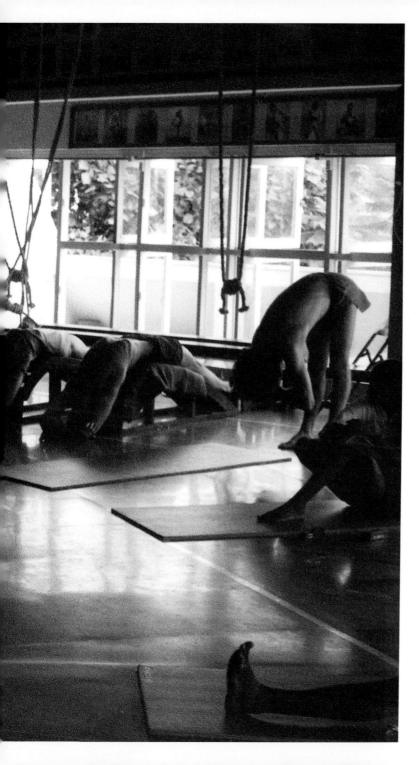

On Fridays, in those early hours of the day when the sun was just rising and the air was still cool, Guruji would set up for backbends. I had heard that Guruji would often do 108 *Urdhva Dhanurasanas*, and so it was.

After very little warming up, sometimes just lying over a bench or chair to open the chest, he would stand in *Tadasana* and completely fluidly, effortlessly would bend, not drop, to take his hands backwards down to the floor without a sound. To come back to *Tadasana* he would alternate between lifting the feet back over his head to come back to *Tadasana* (*Viparita Chakrasana*) or he would stand back up, as if gravity had no pull on him and he was entirely weightless. Effortless effort.

His face was impassive yet focused, and he hardly moved his feet from his original position. You would not have known if he was doing number 5 or number 50. The backbend had that steady flow that displayed no signs of wavering, or fatigue.

We were enthralled by what we saw. The qualities I witnessed in his practice, that full absorption that was so clear even to our beginners eyes, have stayed with me ever since.

PL

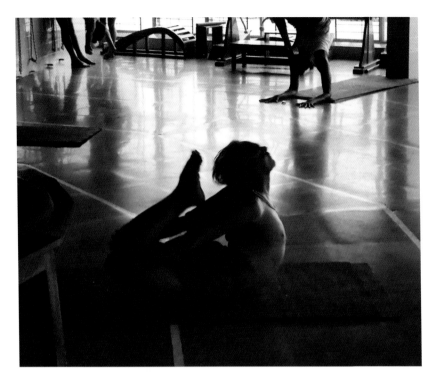

One day I went to the Institute early in the morning near dawn. I don't remember if I was the only person there besides Guruji, but I felt like I was. I was sitting on the steps and all the photos were around the room. The silence was profound. The silence of him working in that room was so still, the stillness of how he was working. The experience I had was almost otherworldly. I sat there and I thought, yes here he is doing all of these *asanas*, but something else is going on underneath all of that. He's doing his practice and it's taking him near God. It's not the physical thing that I'm looking at. I'm looking at something transcending that. It was tasting the spirituality of the practice in the silence. He was present in something profound in what he was doing.

CC

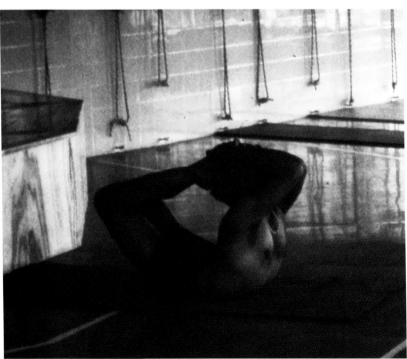

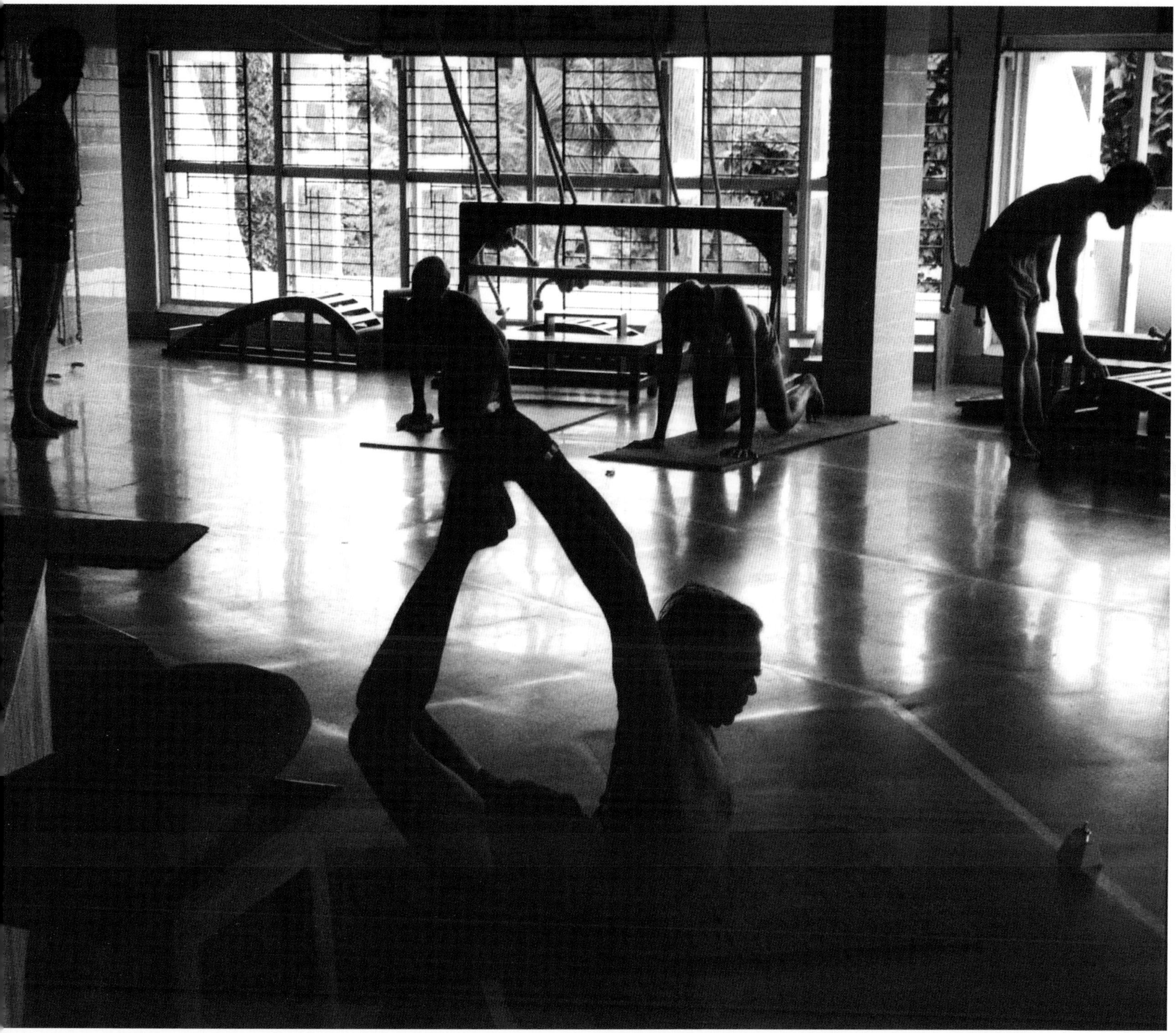

Geetaji

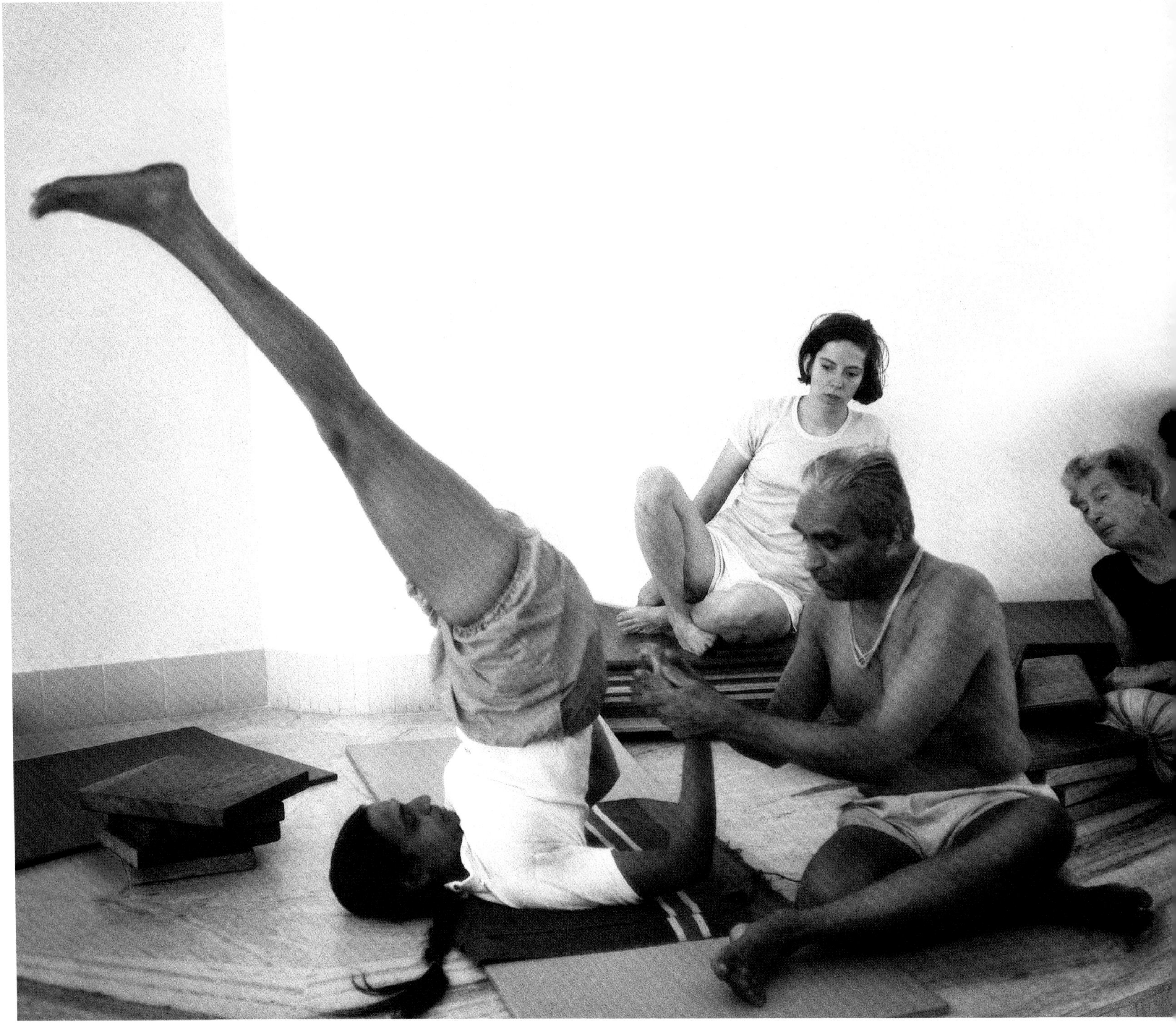

What was significant is that she was very faithfully receiving sacred and special teachings from her father and transferring them. This is how knowledge in India has been preserved and passed on over the centuries.

SC

Geeta was very, very sincere and dedicated in her practice. Her practice was always very diligent. There were times when Guruji gave demonstrations. Those were a piece of art. He was in front and Geeta was a short distance behind him. And not a word was shared. He did not say the name of the *asana*. Only by his breath—his exhalation breath—did she look and follow. It was spectacular.

NK

While teaching, her instructions were clear and precise, her demonstrations enviable. Outside of class I found her to be amicable and friendly. In her stern demeanour, I have always found her eyes to be soft and compassionate. Once, when she realised that I always hesitated to approach her, she told me that I could reach out to her anytime without hesitation. That made me feel as if there was a bond sealed between us.

FAR

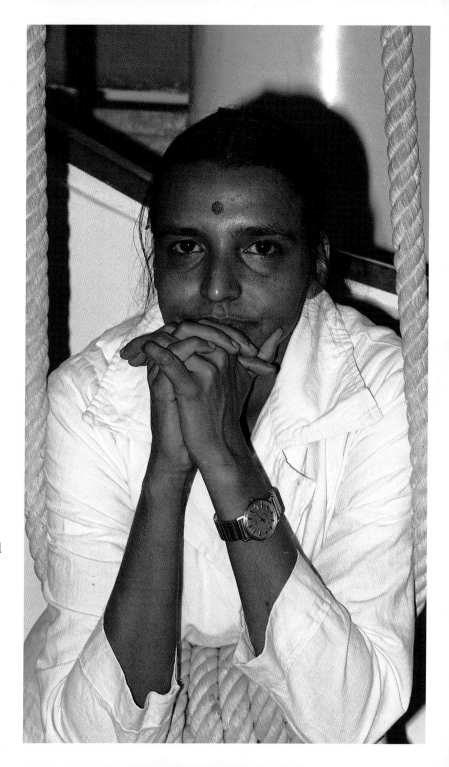

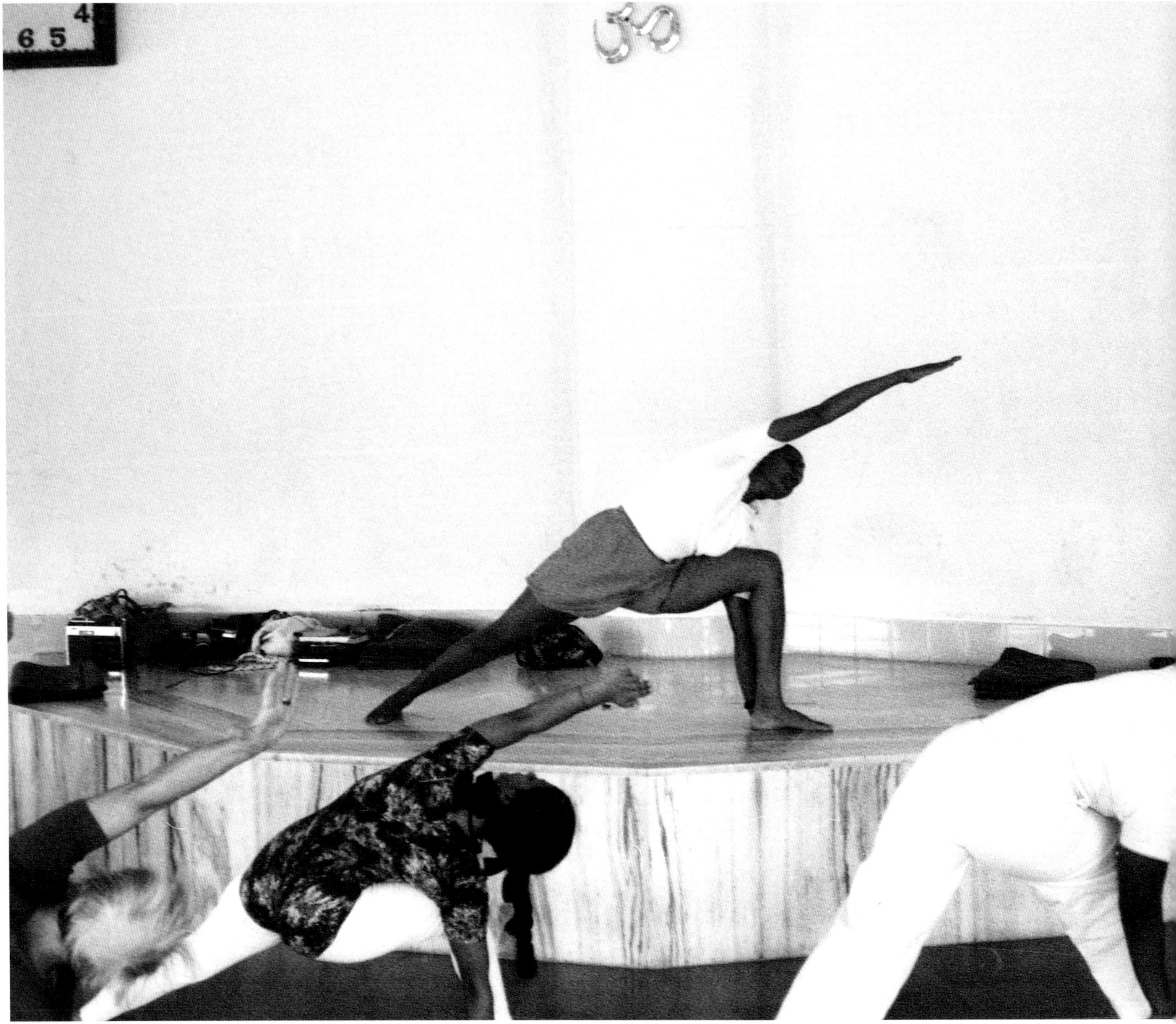

She started with us as a young lanky girl. She was called out of the class by Guruji. We didn't know at first that she was Guruji's daughter. We thought that she must have been an old student to be able to do the *asanas* as Guruji wanted. But she was his daughter and I didn't know that. Guruji made her do *Trikonasana* to show us. "Come on, show them" and gave her one smack—thin, lanky thing! But she stood the smack so well, she stood still and she did the *asana* so gracefully. And then people started talking, saying this is Guruji's daughter. She was very simple and unpretentious from the very beginning and had no unnecessary ego. Yet she was strict like the father.

CD

I remember considering Geetaji as our role model in yoga. Tall and slim, she carried herself with dignity. For me, who was in my early twenties, Geeta was the person to follow. It was later that I realised that her stern exterior was a shield required by the young lady as she set out in the world to teach yoga. In those days of the '70s, the field of yoga was a man's world and as a young and attractive woman, she needed to send the correct message to the men she taught. It was clear that she meant business!

FAR

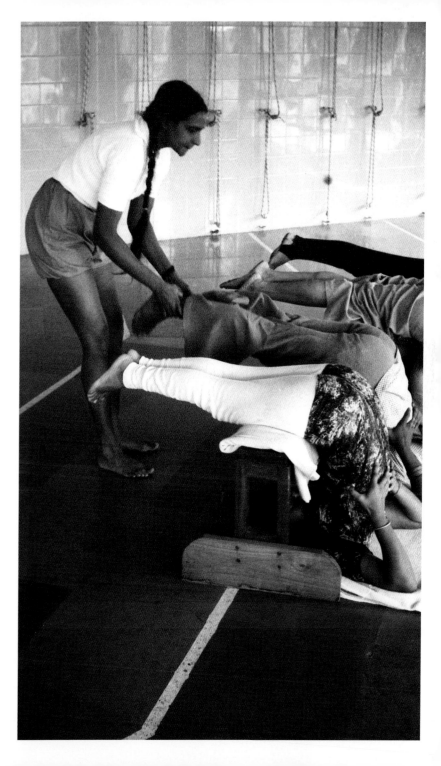

Geetaji was always so powerful in her words, tone and vision from the earliest days. She was omnipresent in the class and her eyes never missed anyone in the hall, no matter how big the class. She often called out to one of us with, "Hey you—green t-shirt!" You might have seen her looking the other way, but you didn't know when she would quickly turn and catch you! Whether you were shy, scared or lazy she ensured that all participated in the class and broke their barriers of fear, stiffness or even social barriers. At that time, when many housewives were very shy, she was so compassionate towards them. She understood what was in the mind of these people. Even after so many decades, it is touching that like Guruji, she still wanted to give and give.

RM

I started going to class when I was very small. I must have been around 7 years old when I was practising in the hall at the Institute one day and my mother, who was also a student at the Institute, came and corrected my *Trikonasana*. Geetaji came over to us right from the other side of the hall and told my mother that "Children should never be corrected. Let them do it on their own. Do not adjust them right now. Let them have the freedom." I was a very small child then. It was important to first have the liking for doing yoga.

AJ

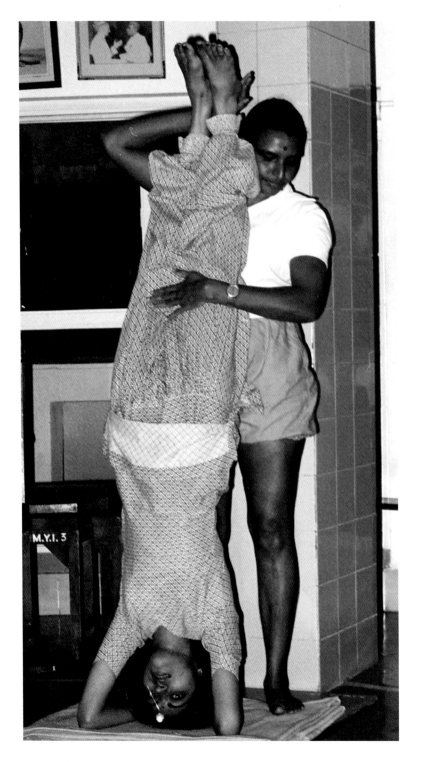

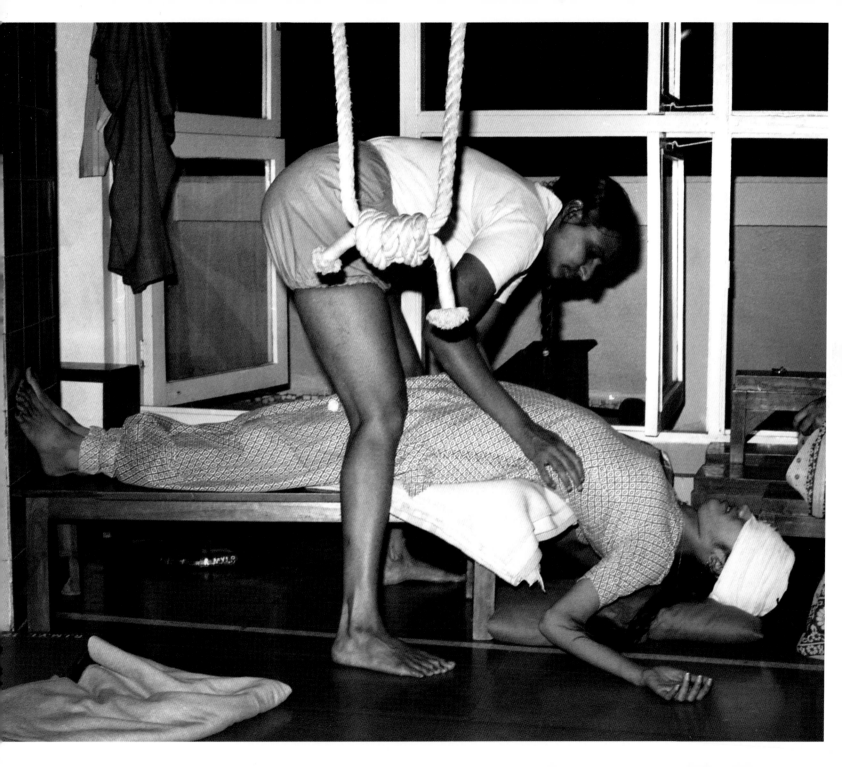

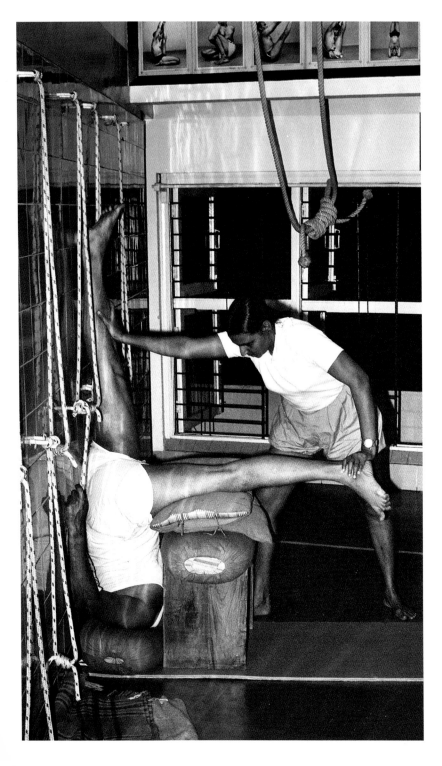

I learned a lot from Geeta conducting the general class. Suddenly in the general class she would start to talk about a particular sort of action that has to come in the pose and it was exactly that action that we were doing, adapting it for somebody in the medical class. I would think about the pose Geeta was instructing us in and start to put together these adaptations. The ways that a pose can change, can target, can really bring its benefit into one principle point or it can be more diffuse. It is catching that which was really the whole global experience of being in Pune. Maybe it does take 20 years to learn that.

As a teacher in the therapy class, she looked into the cases. I mean really looked into the cases. She noticed and she brought concern to those causes, she noticed the changes, the transformations that were not obvious to us, and then she turned her concern to the revelation that we did not see. She revealed our ignorance to us.

SQ

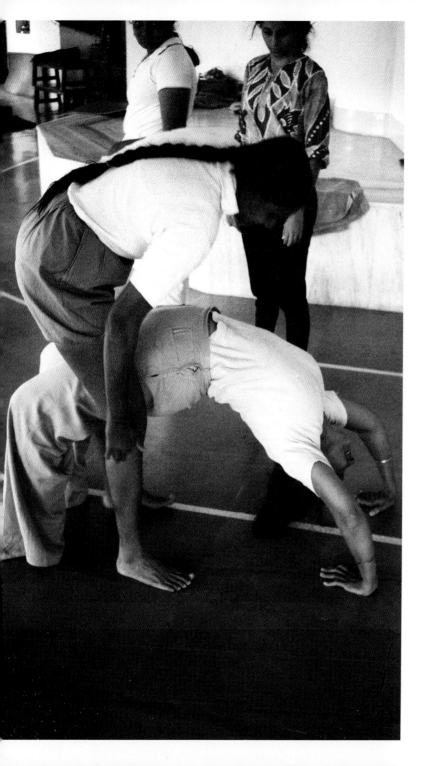

Geeta was always a fiery teacher, right from the beginning. Anyone could see that she was the daughter of BKS Iyengar! The same fire and passion for the subject of yoga. No one would be spared a sharp reprimand for mistakes which were unacceptable. She was a no-nonsense person, working hard to bring relief to the suffering of students in the therapy class. It had always been to her a matter of great importance that the suffering of her students must be overcome. No effort was enough, nor considered a waste in that direction. As she was a student of Indian philosophy, she wove her knowledge of the philosophy of yoga through her teaching. Her compassion was always genuine and as an individual she was then and is now hugely loved by her students.

FAR

After studying with another teacher in India for a few years I finally realised I had to study with the Iyengars. When I arrived for the first time at the Institute in 1976 I went and knocked on the front door of the Iyengars' house. They told me that Guruji was away teaching in South Africa and I should go up to the hall and see Geeta. I went to the hall and she was the only one in the room doing her practice. I felt I couldn't disturb her, but after I sat there quietly for some time she called me over. I introduced myself and she said, "Come tonight to the class at 6 p.m." It was a *Pranayama* class and I remember instantly feeling that this was exactly what I had been missing. I felt like I had come home. From the very first class of her inspiring and powerful teaching I knew I was in the right place.

JP

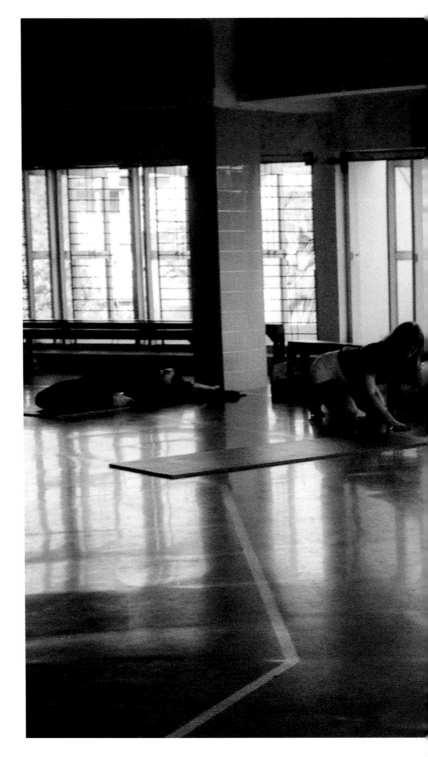

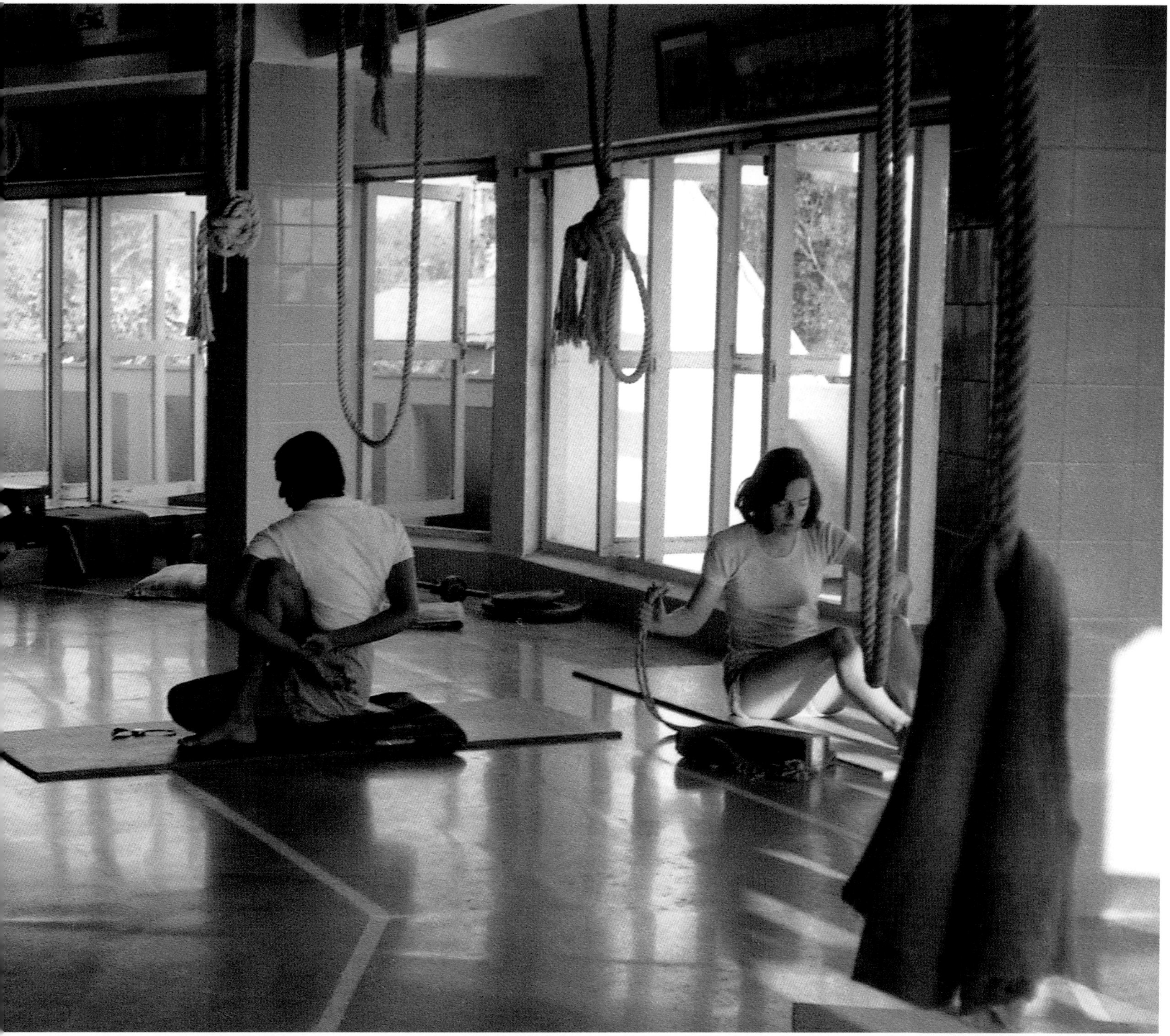

Prashantji

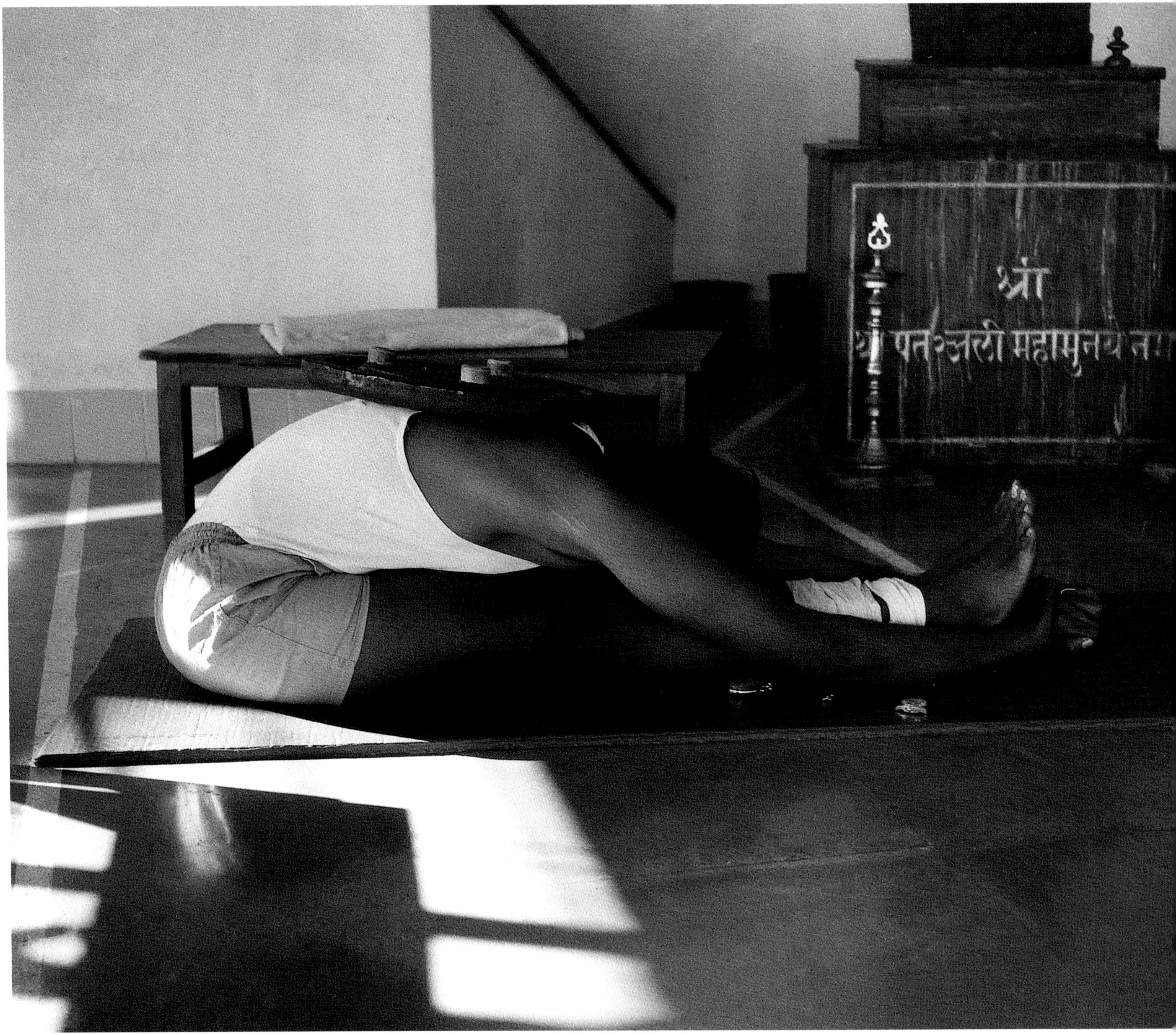
श्री
पतञ्जली महामुनये

Guruji would visit Mumbai on every weekend and later, Geetaji or Prashantji would come on alternate weekends. I was in my teens and whenever there was a *Pranayama* class, we youngsters were asked to do backbends, rope work or abdominal *asanas*. The rest of the class was 'sleeping' as far as we were concerned. We did part of the general class and while they did *Pranayama*, we were asked to do these different *asanas*. We had to stay for many counts—multiples of 50 in the same *asana*— like *Urdhva Prasarita Padasana* or *Urdhva Dhanurasana*; sometimes it was very fast movement; sometimes it was slow motion. It was so challenging and the body would ache for 2-3 days but we would look forward to these classes. Later when Prashantji had the accident, it was so touching when he continued to help each one of us do *Viparita Chakrasana* from the platform at RIMYI. Although one elbow was broken he continued helping each of us with one hand. Each of the 80 students was individually helped by him. He would be so fast, it was impossible to keep up with him. Later, I realised that it was through this swiftness, that he was making us overcome all the *antarayas*—obstacles that Patanjali refers to in the 30th *sutra* of the first chapter—we managed to overcome disease, dullness, laziness, doubt, lack of perseverance, maintaining and going beyond whatever was achieved. As he often says now, "Yoga begins much later."

RM

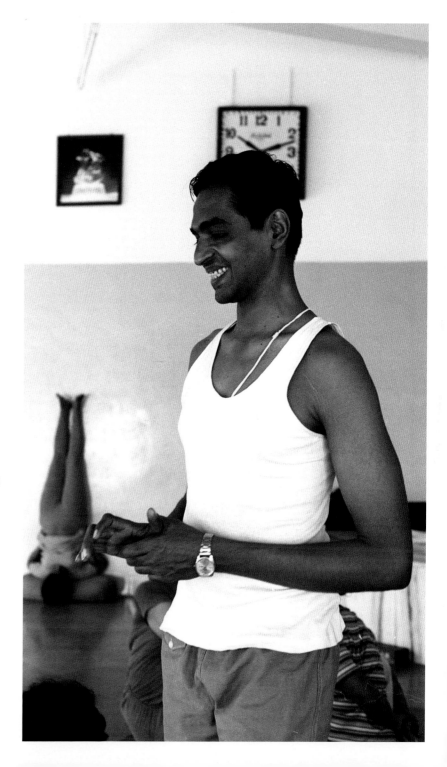

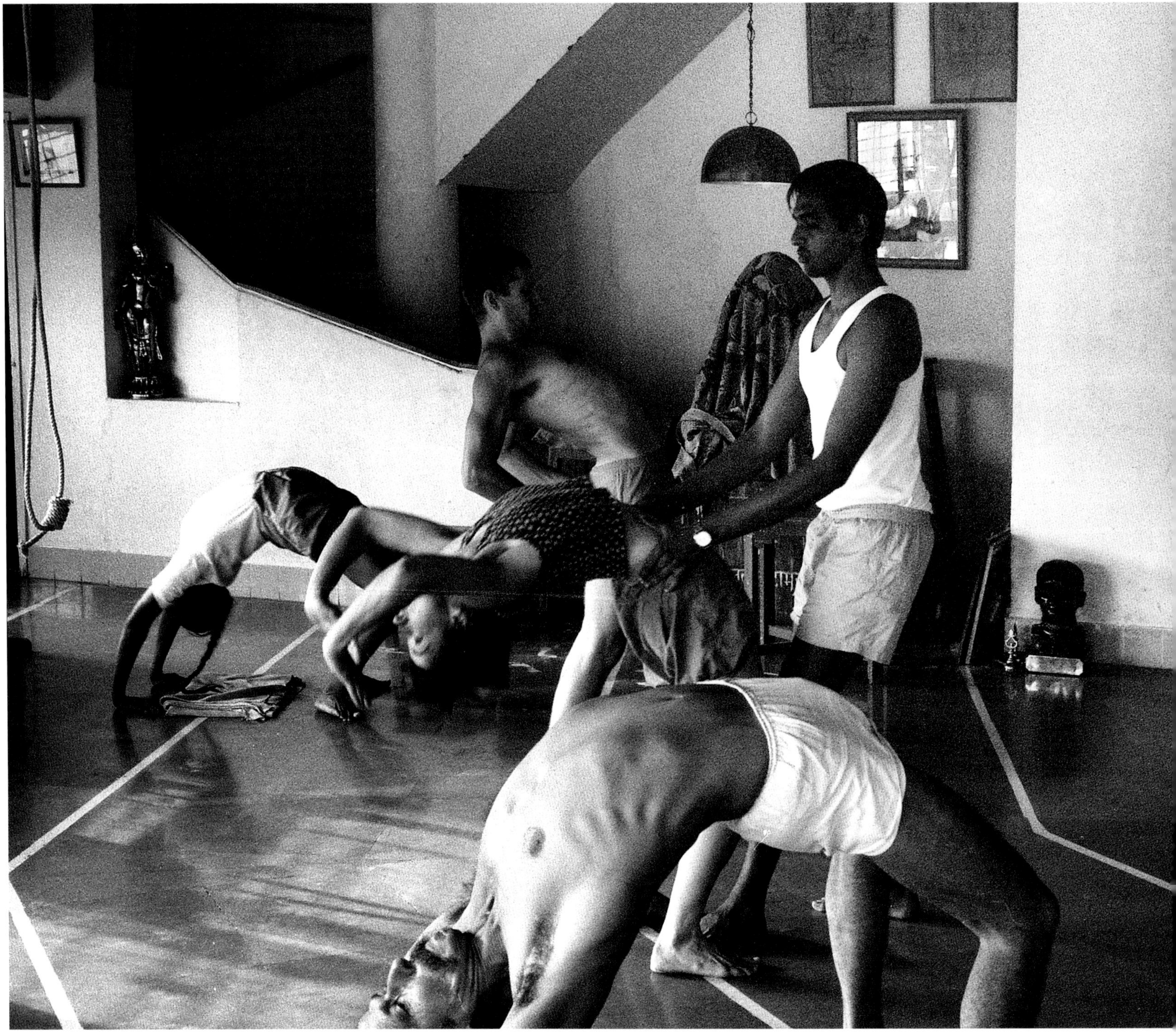

My first meeting with Prashant, as we would address him those days, was in Mumbai, in the Saturday afternoon class. It was a class usually taught by Guruji.

That weekend, Guruji did not come and instead Prashant had come to teach. Since I was pretty new to that class and not knowing who he was, I was a bit apprehensive. I soon realised that my apprehension was uncalled for. This young man taught a very powerful class with firm instructions. At first it appeared to me as if he was dispassionate in his instructions and not really interested in whether they were being followed. I very soon found that to be a mistaken perception when I was swiftly corrected with the flick of a hand or a foot to surprisingly find myself in a more balanced and lighter condition! I still remember the feeling I had in that elevated *Sarvangasana*!

Later when I started visiting Pune, I got to understand Prashantji better. I found him to be soft and compassionate within. Those days I was a student and keen on philosophy. I found that Prashantji had a lot of knowledge of philosophy and particularly yoga philosophy. I was very impressed by his vast amount of knowledge and the volumes of reading and his phenomenal memory.

I remember that in those days after the evening Pranayama class he would proceed to the library with a small group of students and discuss the yoga sutras. Back then, there would be only 4 or 5 of us who were interested in such learning. I still remember his handwritten notes which he would generously allow me to take to read. It is these notes which are now being turned into valuable books of knowledge and wisdom.

I remember Prashantji's accident and how even then he taught all of us a lesson about how to look at life unfazed, without a single word of regret or self-pity for what had happened—no frustration, no dejection—his body needed mending but the person, Prashant, continued on his journey of Yoga finding his own ways of continuing with his practices. Gradually his teachings became more philosophical, his language developed its own vocabulary and his teaching its own style.

FAR

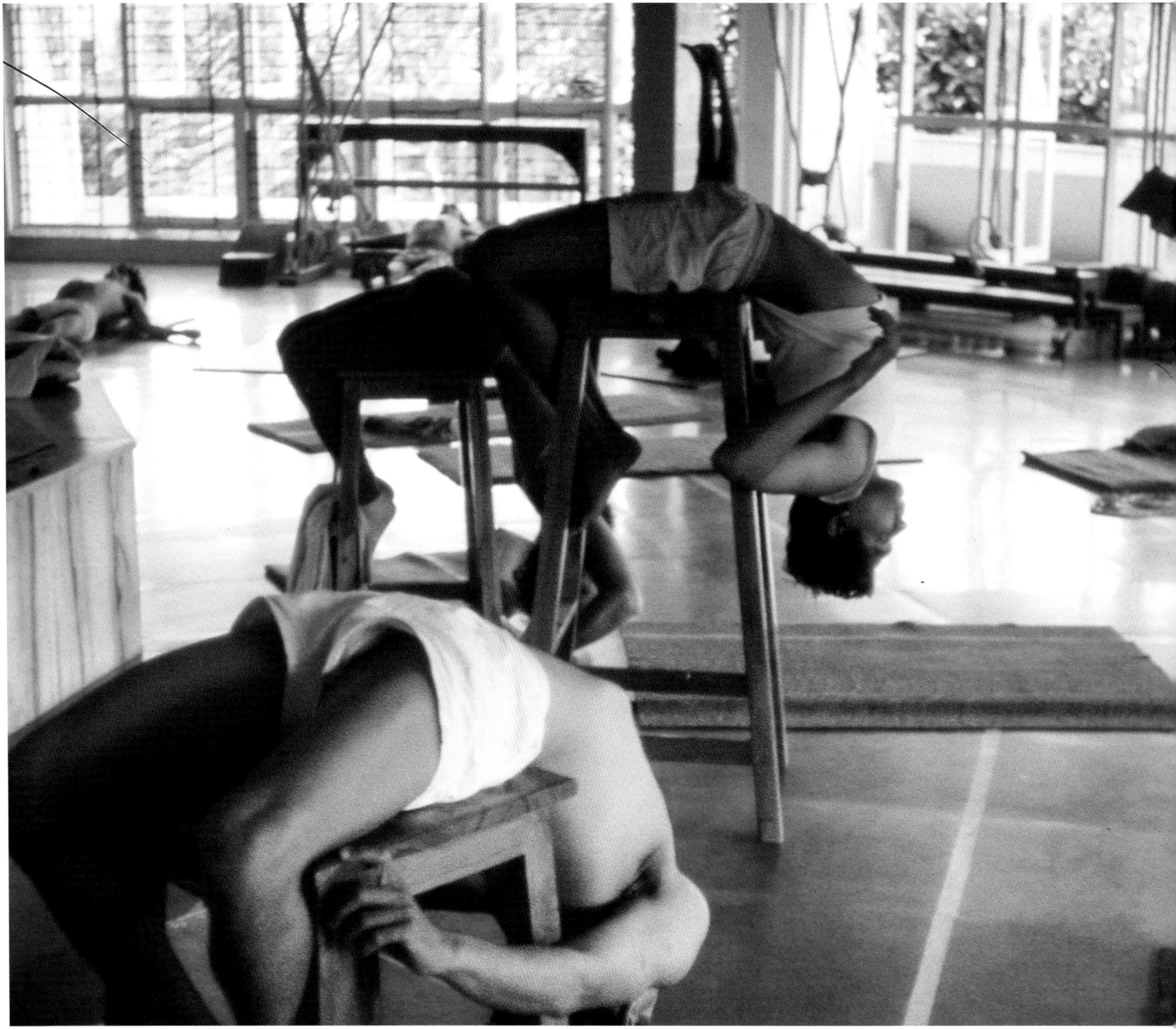

Prashant's popularity amongst young people was phenomenal. Do I recall correctly that once when he came on to the stage we were all chanting "Prashant! Prashant! Prashant!" I am ever grateful that he allowed my wee children into his classes in the main hall and launched them on their yoga journey: They recall that he would ask them to hang on the ceiling rope, and then he would wind up the rope, and then when he released the rope the kids would be spinning round and round! It is admirable that he made this time and effort. He continues to reach out to pupils and has evolved into an unmatchable commentator on the practice, philosophy and culture of yoga.

SC

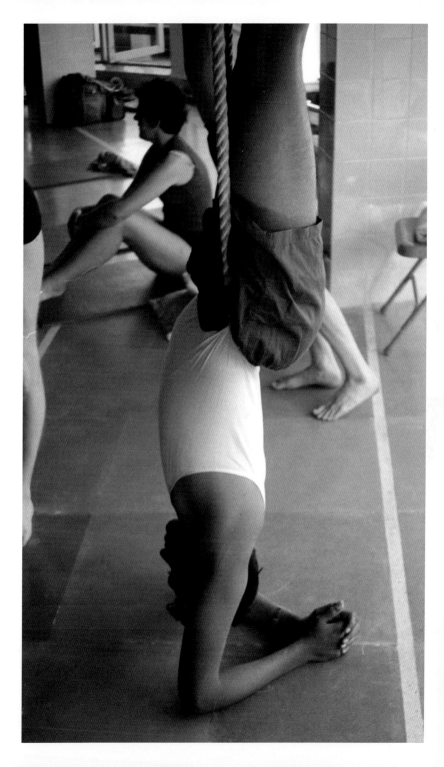

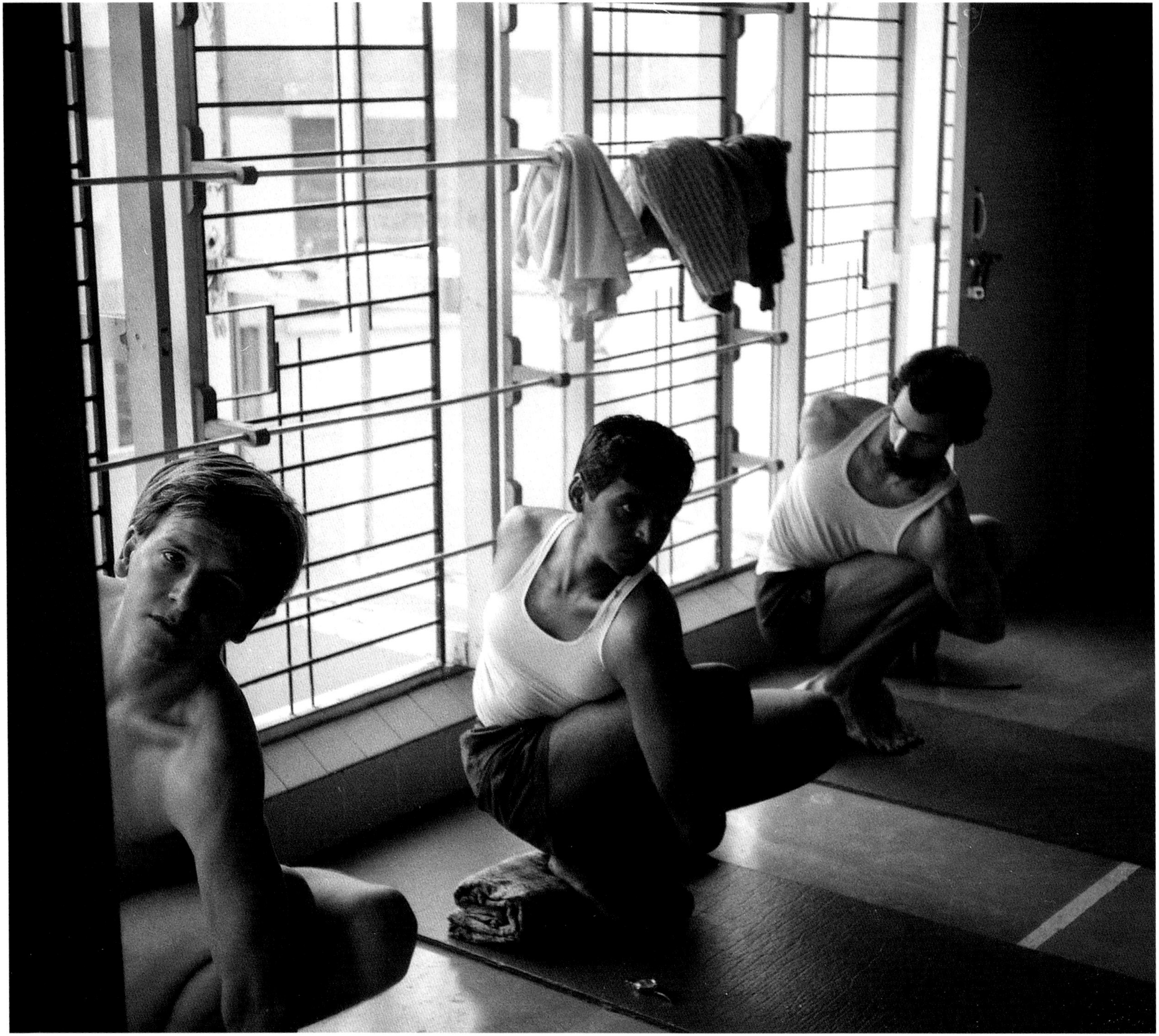

I went to the Institute in the early days one morning and for some reason things had been cancelled. I went into the hall and Prashant was alone in the room practising. He was doing handstand, dropping over and standing up—*Viparita Chakrasana*. He was blindfolded. I was there for a long time and then left. He must have done 108. That was a special memory from those days.

KP (Kay Parry)

When I would enter the class in the '70s, I remember there was often one person doing very difficult poses behind the column. I particularly remember him doing *Ardha Matsyendrasana*. Interestingly, after the 2 hour class finished I would just have a peek at this person practising there and he was still in *Ardha Matsyendrasana*. At that time we didn't know it was Guruji's son Prashant.

RN

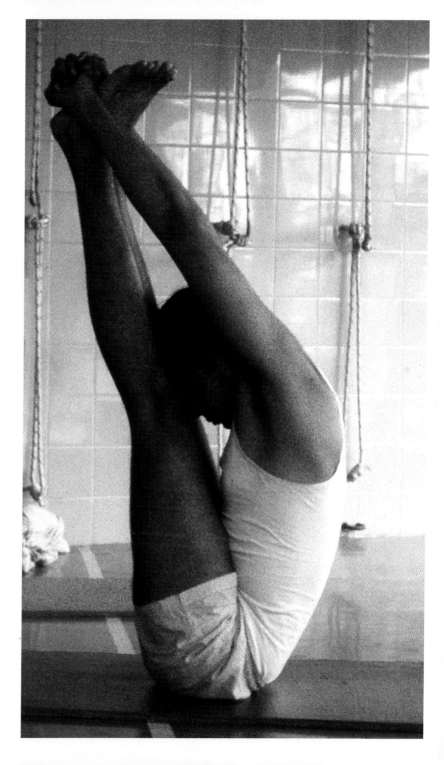

The Medical Classes

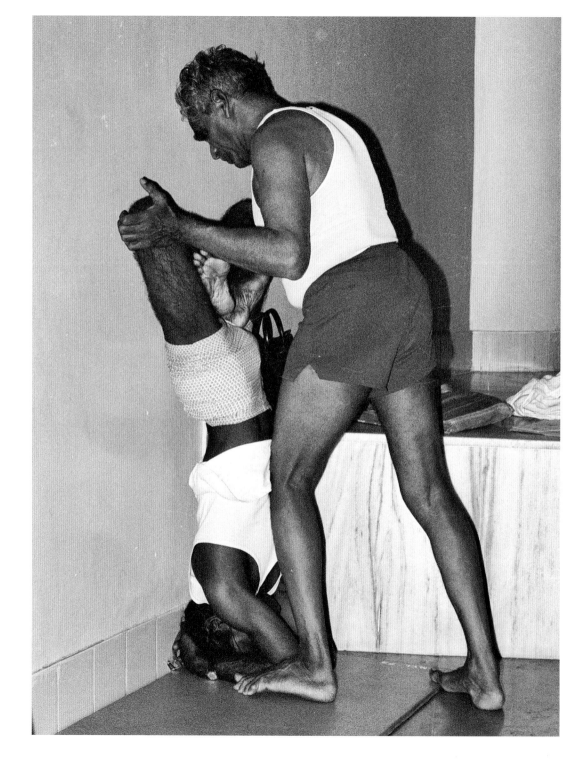

Wonder and astonishment. These are the emotions those who observed or assisted Guruji and Geetaji in the medical classes at RIMYI experienced. As you will read, they helped countless students with their health issues in such an exceptional way. Students came to the classes with unique problems, sometimes even those that were untreatable by the medical profession. Once, Guruji revealed that he had never worked with a particular case before, but you would not have known that in the class. He worked with such supreme confidence, utilising experimentation until he achieved the desired effect for the student.

He would often ask how the student felt, but their verbal response was not how Guruji intuited that the effect was correct or not. He would observe their skin, the clenching around the outer corner of the eye, how they breathed, how the internal layers of the body were connecting. If a student gave him a long list of problems, he would not necessarily work directly on those problems, but perhaps, he addressed the depression that he could see despite it not being listed. Despite the chaos that permeated the medical classes, Guruji would know from the opposite side of the room (with his back turned away!) whether an assistant was adjusting the student in the pose incorrectly. In the process of helping the students, Guruji helped the assistants improve as well.

LS (Lois Steinberg)

In a way it's not really well-known or understood just how important the medical class was for Guruji. Perhaps you had to either be an assistant in the class or a patient to even try to grasp what he was doing. He was even more intense in the medical class and gave so much of himself. He had such an enquiring and penetrating mind like no other and in the challenge of the problems he came to solutions that no one else could see. It was often uncanny how he could figure these things out. It seemed unbelievable except that we were there seeing and experiencing it. He wanted to help the people so they could progress in their lives and in yoga and he gave his all. The number of people he helped is incalculable. It was way beyond being generous. It was something else.

JP

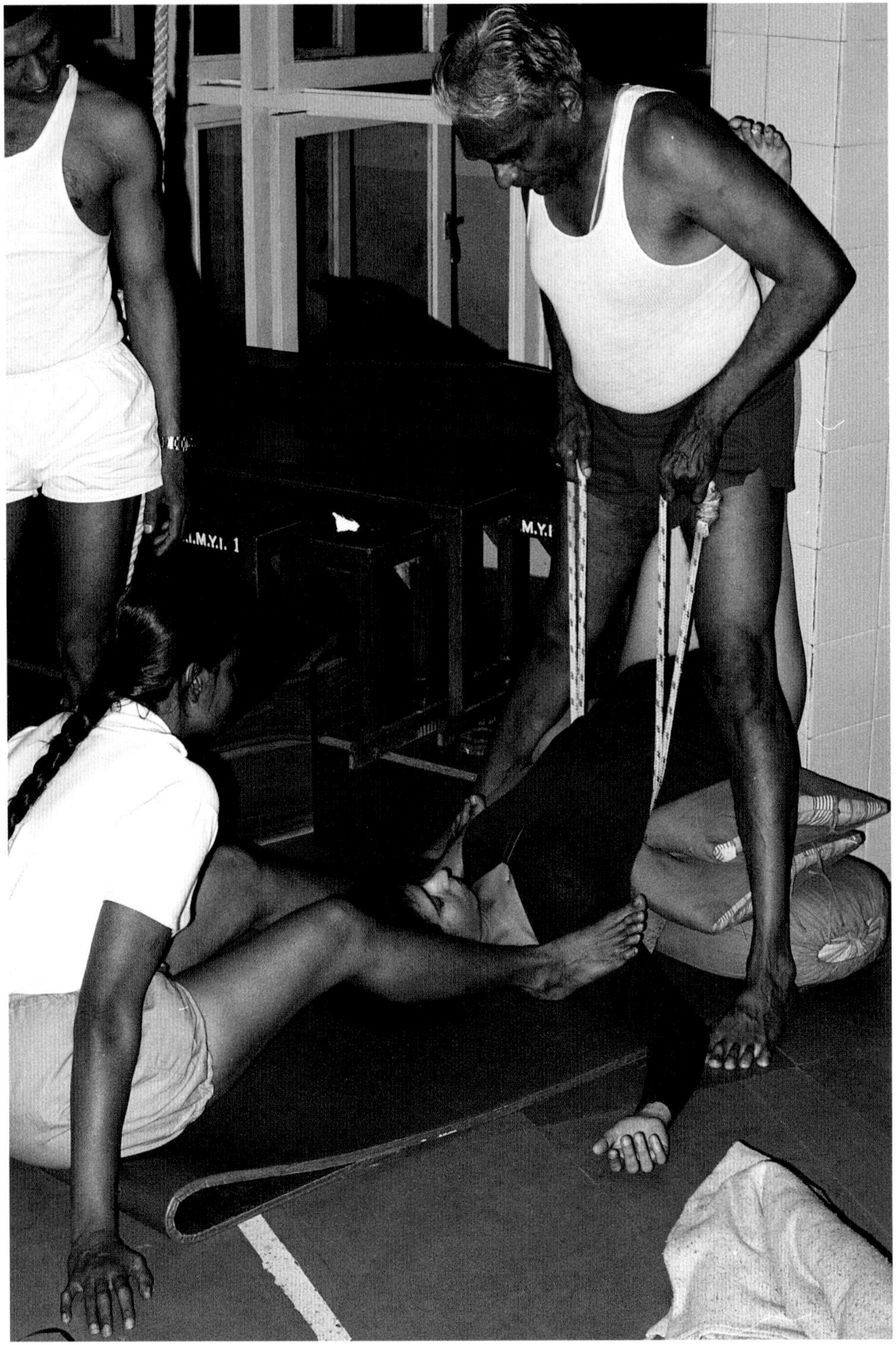
M.Y.I. 1
M.Y.I

The moment Geeta and Guruji stepped into the therapy class—the energy of the room lit up, and it was something to watch them both in action, quite unique, quite extraordinary. It was breath catching.

Before I left for Pune, I asked my teacher if should I tell them about my injured foot, and she said to me, "You can tell them if you like, but they will know everything there is to know about your foot by the time you've crossed the hall."

Working with Guruji in the beginning was terrifying. I had no idea what was going on, which meant I couldn't guess what might be needed. So the instructions of what to do didn't always even make any sense, because for me there was no context. Guruji was using his own language of what had to be done and you had to be very fast and read any clue as to what was to be done. You were constantly working at the edge of yourself.

There is one aspect that everyone knows of Guruji and that is as the conductor of classes, how his voice holds you in. He takes you into a place and he really does transport a whole class. He has harnessed the power of the speech. He is a master of that—timing, rhythm, tone, choice of words. But when working with him in the medical class he would often give almost cryptic instructions, obscure instructions, from which you're meant to know what is needed. Yet, he himself didn't dialogue a lot, in fact, hardly at all apart from those cryptic instructions. On reflection what I realise is a lot of the lesson to be learned was that in working directly on people in that medical situation it is really you. You are working from a deep place inside you. It's not a place where you broadcast. I really do believe that

is why he didn't dialogue a lot. Working with him, you had to learn quickly. Of course he did repeat the work day in and day out on the person and alter it slowly over a period of time. You had to realise quickly what was needed for this pose and you had to really remember if he was going to do the same pose the next day. You really had to remember exactly what belt was tied in what direction, which little bit of spacer to put where, the subtle differences required.

And what I realised then, big clue, was his process of working medically is actually non-vocal. It's not technical; it doesn't matter how many times you photograph a pose; it doesn't matter how much medical knowledge you have, how much anatomy you have. The real healing work is totally beyond speech and that's where he is working from in himself. That's why he didn't dialogue that much while you're working with him. But if you were waiting to be told what this art of therapy was, forget it. None of the Iyengars will explain that to you.

SQ

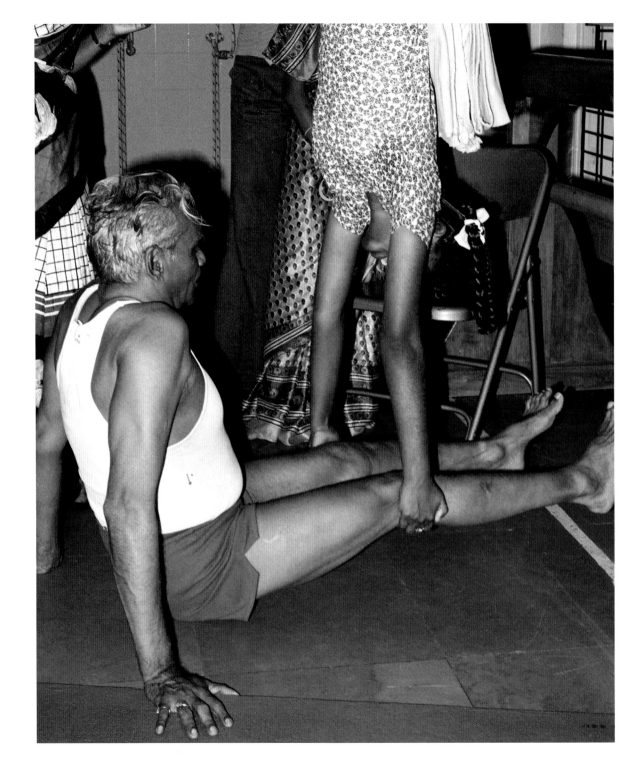

144

I remember a particular instance—it's not that he taught me something about a condition and what to take for it—but he taught me something about the human condition that arrives at discomfort, ill ease, that arrives at physical/physiological conditions. One was a girl who was suffering from dysmenorrhoea, very painful periods. It was quite interesting because she was doing some basic work in therapy class, being looked after. Guruji came up to her, and he said, "Look at her face. Look at how unhappy she is." And she did look quite unhappy, and she looked a little bit afraid as well, I thought. How he treated her was no different from what he taught for somebody with deep endogenous depression; he didn't particularly apply the *asanas* to help with dysmenorrhoea. And her menstruation returned to normal and it stopped being so painful for her.

It gave me an insight into the belief system that they're coming from. It's so inevitable that we will try to overlay our scientific medical model. We are looking for clues of what to do and we are looking through the lens of our already existing knowledge of what we've learned so far; we've been educated in the scientific analytic model. What he's looking at and what he treated was embodiment of consciousness because there actually isn't a difference between the mental frame and the physiological body.

He had a funny thing he'd like to say, as a joke, he would say, "I'm a learner, I'm just a learner", and then he'd say, "but I'm not a beginner". He was naturally very, very curious with a very youthful, inquiring mind. He had a fascination and a delight in learning and he always wanted to "find out", and I think that drove him a lot. I think he was very interested in his own learning process. Certain cases were coming to him and the penetration of understanding that was required for him to reach in and help that student was quite different. It was a field of his own *Sadhana*, and just gave him a different look into his own *Sadhana*. In some ways having to solve those cases meant he had to call on a much deeper experience within his own *Sadhana*, and that essentially his therapeutic work and his practice were linked, they were not separate things. They were giving him something in his own growth because of what he was needing to reach into, to find the solution for someone.

SQ

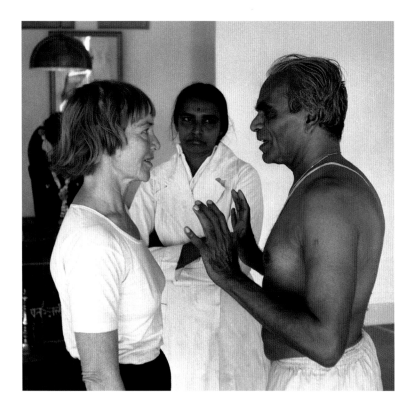
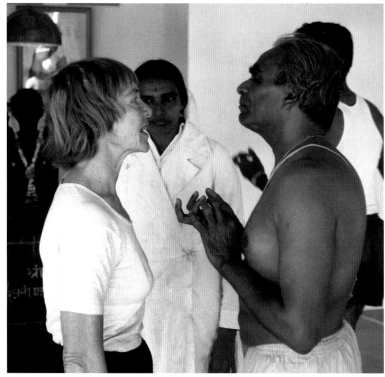

This was an old friend of Guruji's from his years of teaching the philosopher J. Krishnamurti. She came for help after suddenly developing marked problems with memory and confusion. I asked him what was wrong with her and he said, "Her *Kundalini* is going the wrong way." He worked intensely with her for several months and the problem disappeared. She had a lasting recovery.

JP

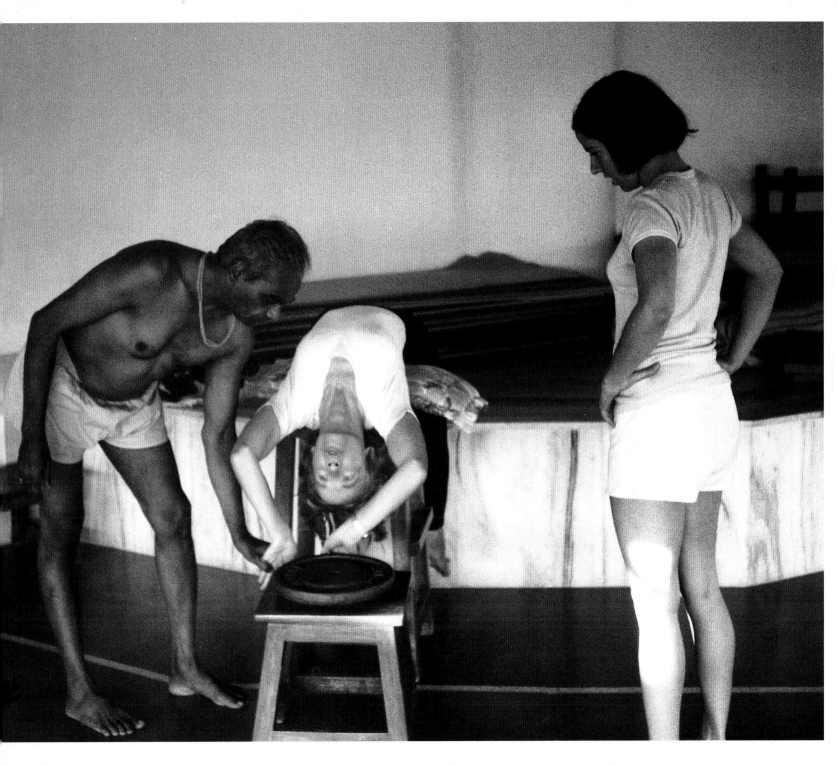

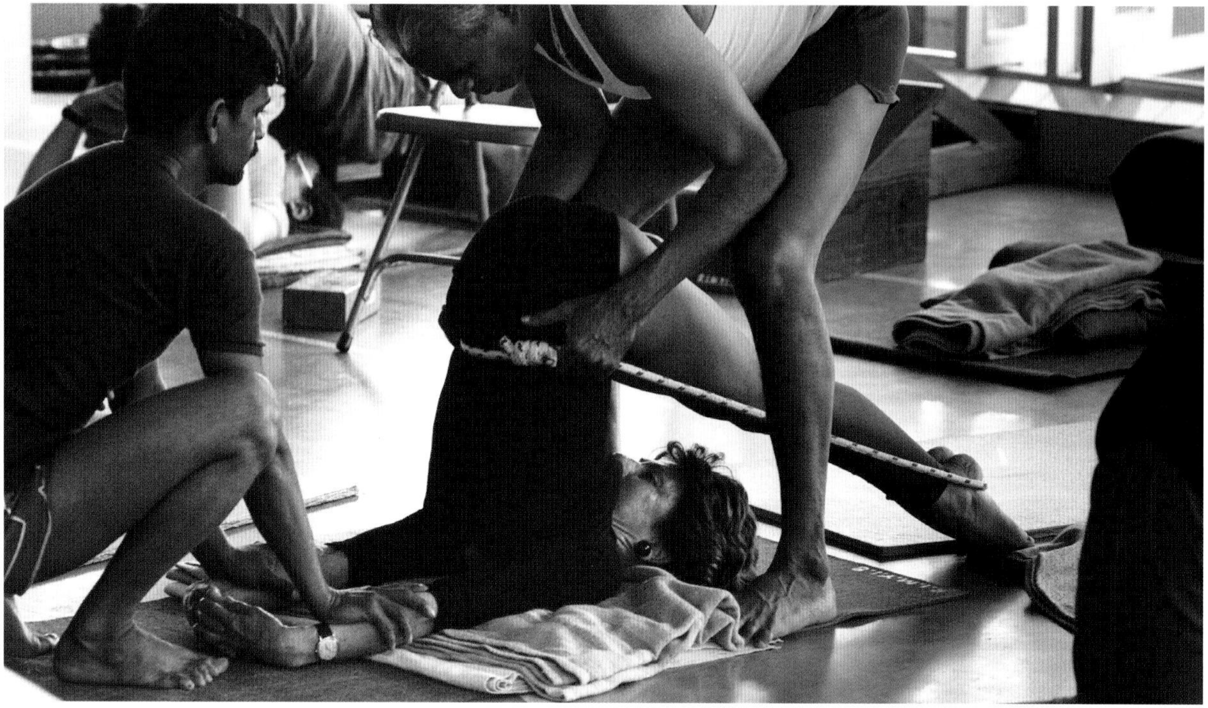

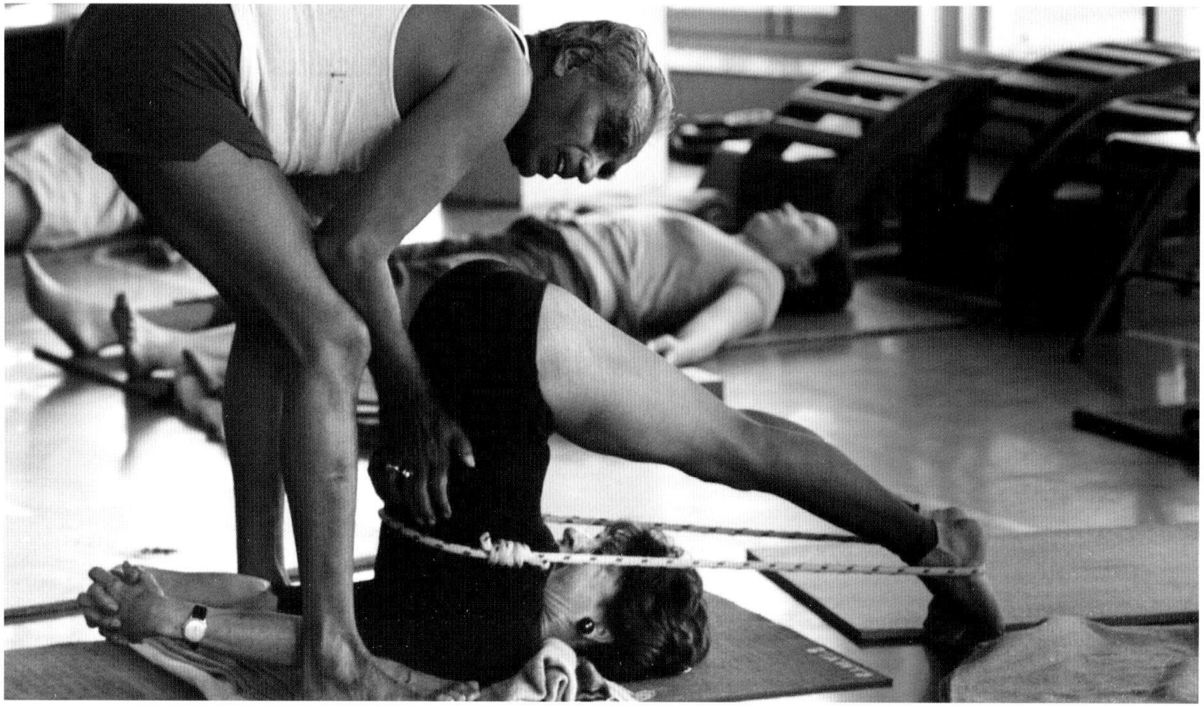

Diligently, I would arrive early and sit on the steps and observe the medical classes. After one month of this, Guruji called me in to help in the medical class. He asked me to help support a paralysed man at the trestle. One of the assistants was being admonished for what he did wrong. Guruji was admonishing him and I took it as an unsaid message to do what you are told in this class. He would say, "If you make a mistake like that again I will hit you twice as hard." He was a genius and could not tolerate others making assumptions. It was difficult, a trial by fire.

To assist in the medical class was not a course for assistants. We were expected to know the classical yoga poses to understand what was going on in the class. I would try the things that were given in medical class on my own body so that I could understand.

I was given a group to teach in the class. They were students using the wall for support. Once I moved the group out to the balcony trying to teach a point in *Parivrtta Trikonasana*. They didn't understand my instructions and were not getting the point. I moved on then to another *asana*. Just after that I felt something hard on the back of my neck, thinking that the back of the window fell on me. It was in fact Guruji giving me a whack on the neck. He instructed that I should never move on to another instruction until the students understood what I was trying to teach them. He insisted that we as teachers must observe the students. I was learning how to look, see, correct, adjust and to use simple words and that has stayed with me until now.

His genius was that he would really see what was wrong with people. He needed a simple yes or no answer to, "Can you feel pain?" from the student. If he received a long list of complaints or explanations that was not actually a response to his question, Guruji would walk away. He did not have time to quell your ego. He wanted to know if something was working or not. You needed to surrender to him wanting to help you. If you surrendered you would get all the help. "You have to wash your brain so I can teach you," he would say.

LS

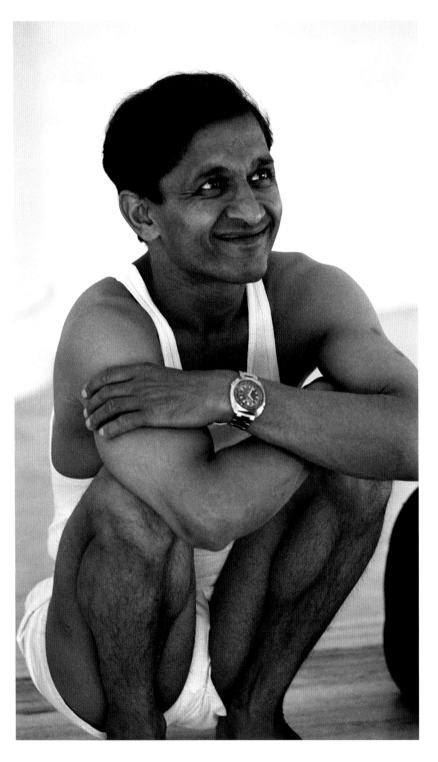

Shah was there from the beginning. Always cheerful and unassuming in his manner, it was a joy to have him assisting in the class and especially in the medical class. You could learn a lot about how to assist with Guruji in the medical class by watching him. He was observant, quickly caught what Guruji wanted him to do and seemed quite free of personal motivation. For decades he was always there, gladly giving of himself for others.

JP

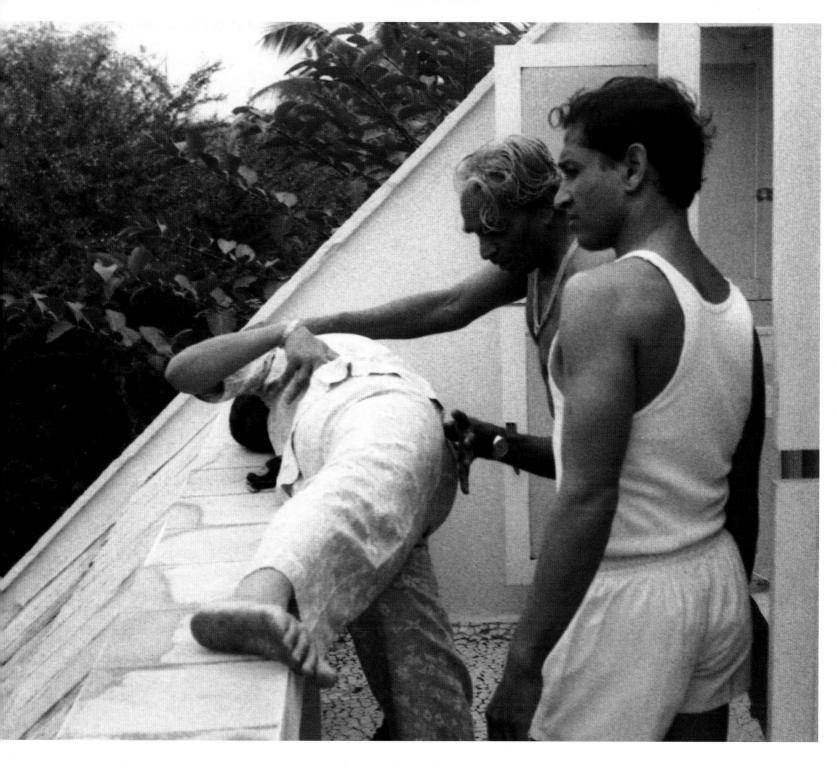

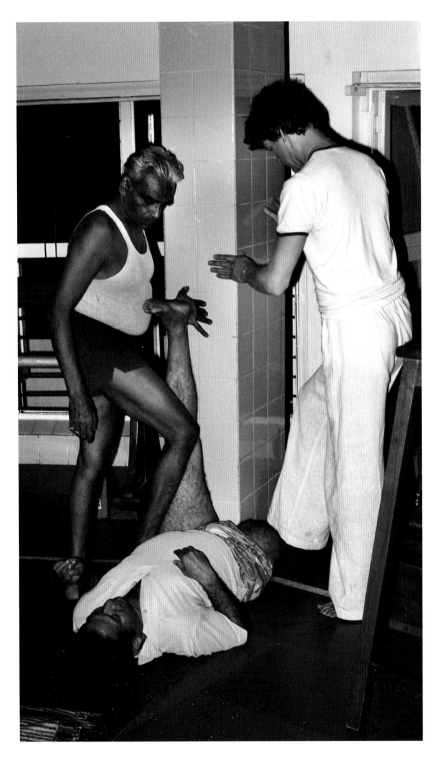

I went to India to search for a yoga teacher to help me with a failed low back operation at the age of 21. I met someone who said if he had my problem, he would go to this man named Iyengar. Eventually I went to his house to meet him and said, "I've got a back problem and I want to be a yoga teacher." He said, "Just like that you want to fix your back and become a yoga teacher? Hmph!" He said he was too busy and to go away. When I then asked if there was anyone else who could help me, he said, "No, I am the only one who can help you." The next thing he said was, "Come back at 4:30 and I will look at you."

I remembered that someone had said that Iyengar had written a book called *Light On Yoga*. I stopped at a large bookshop and when I opened up the book and saw the photos I was completely stunned. This guy could do anything. He had to know his body completely and he must be able to show me how to use mine and cure my problem.

I went back in the afternoon and he looked at me and asked, "So you have been doing yoga, have you? Show me." I told him I'd been doing yoga from a book but had stopped due to pain. "Useless! Hopeless! Pathetic!" were his words while I went through the motions of Salute to the Sun. Then he said, "Do this." And he did *Trikonasana*. I looked at him in disbelief and said, "Are you kidding me mate?" But I did as instructed and lunged into *Trikonasana*—BOOM—down I went, yelling in pain. He said, "Get up! What are you doing?!" He then instructed me to go to one of the windows with vertical steel bars. He had a piece of rope and wrapped it around the bars and holding it, raised one leg and lifted his chest, telling me, "Do this." Again, I thought he must be joking. I tried, but I had no flexibility in my legs. Eventually with him instructing me, "Do this! Do that! Not that, this!" I experienced something I had not experienced in 3 years. Relief from pain!

PD (Peter Davies)

One year I was frustrated with a pain in my shoulder and made arrangements to go to Pune. I had not told Guruji why I was there, but when he saw me he asked "What is your problem?" I had the chance to join the medical class and I had the honour to receive his help for every single *asana*. This was a total transformation in my practice. I thought I was giving my best, but with his help I reached a new level. This has remained for me a lesson in intensity and surrender for the rest of my life.

GG

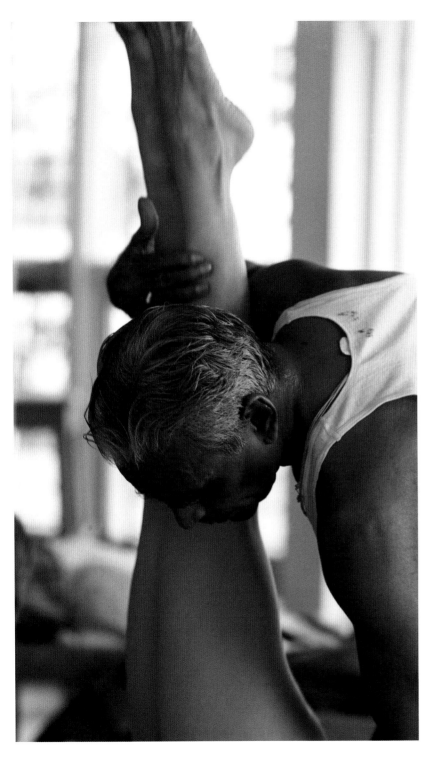

After a traumatic spinal injury, surgeons informed me that I faced paralysis even if I had a lumbar fusion operation. The injury was so severe that they told me that I could be in a wheelchair for the rest of my life. In my worst moment, I remembered Guruji working with patients when I was at RIMYI in 1976 that he called his "hopeless cases". My hope was renewed! I too was a hopeless case and knew he was the one person in the world who could save me. Friends helped me escape the hospital and I set out for Pune. Guruji's subtle and delicate adjustments gradually reinserted my vertebrae back into my spinal column over several months. Then, intensely working under his direct guidance, Guruji took me from the invalid stage, to getting back onto my feet, to walking again and to difficult *asanas* in only 6 months.

My spine was made erect again and I avoided paraplegia. When it came time to leave, I feared my spine would fall apart again when sitting on the long flight home without Guruji watching over me directly. Guruji listened consolingly to my concern and with great excitement, hatched a plan. He said he had to find a deck chair that was shaped like an airplane seat and told me to come back that evening. He was ready for me with the chair when I got back and we did *Paripurna Navasana* with my feet against a wall in the RIMYI courtyard. It required a full stretch of my spine and sciatic nerves. Guruji showed me that I was restored to my former limberness and could do what I feared most. It was Guruji's miraculous wisdom to work on my fear. While showing me the "plane chair yoga" he was also trying to get me to laugh. He was so funny but also a magician. He was the magic. He was the harbinger of hope. He told me, "Your pain will disappear

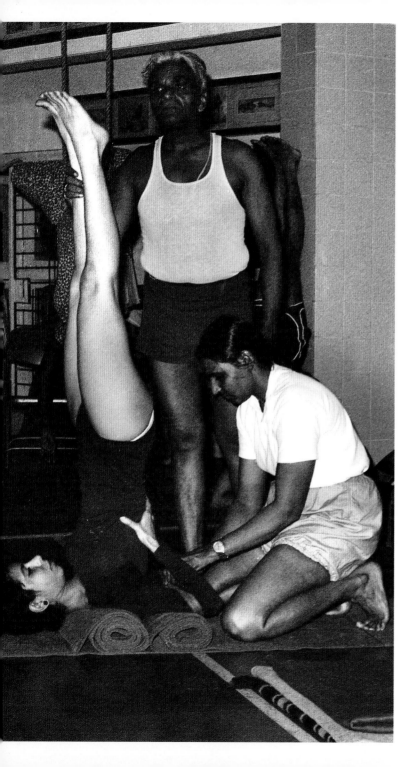

in 3 days time once you rest on a soft bed in the U.K. at your brother's house." The next day, on board my flight with the set of plane poses he prescribed, I sat during takeoff and other intervals with my feet against the headrest of the seat in front of me. *Paripurna Navasana* helped to keep my spine from locking as did standing, twisting and backbending *asanas*. I also did headstand and shoulderstand in the back of the plane. I have been fine since the 3 days after I left Pune. Exactly as Guruji said. That was in 1980.

EH (Evlaleah Howard)

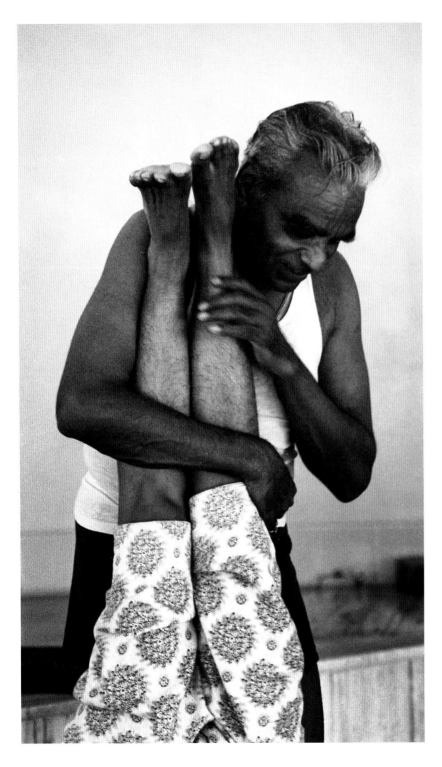

I think that everyone has suffering in life at some point or another. I often think of Guruji as the lifeboat that shows us how to go from suffering to the opposite shore.

During those years in my 30s I was in and out of depression. I never talked to Guruji about it. Guruji assigned me to help a woman in medical class with depression. Intense backbendings, arm balances, dropping back. I think that Guruji knew that I was suffering from depression and this was his way of helping me. I felt that he chose me for her because she had the same thing. He saw everything, but he didn't always say what he saw. It was very very powerful that he would choose me at that age to work with someone.

PW

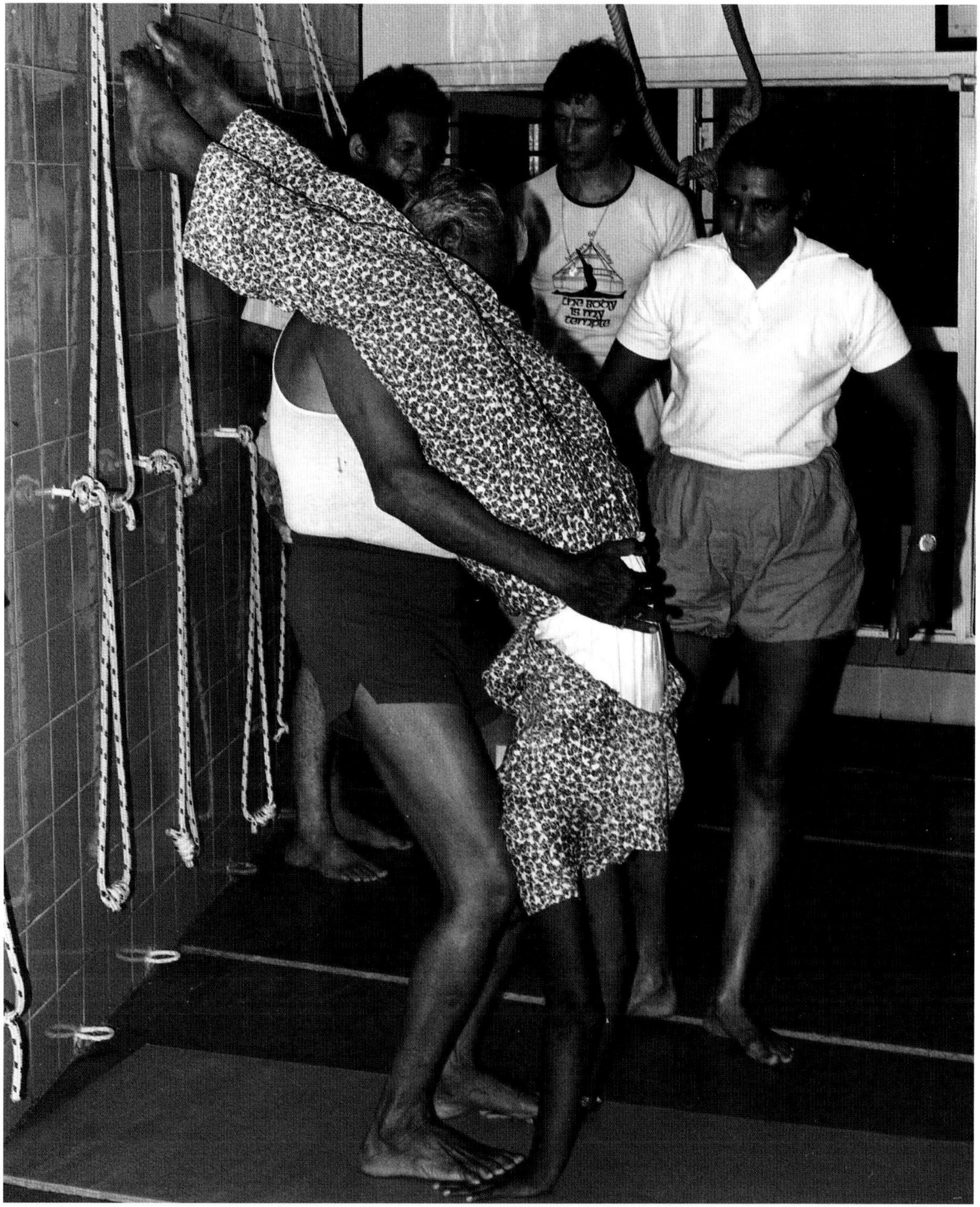
the body
is my
temple

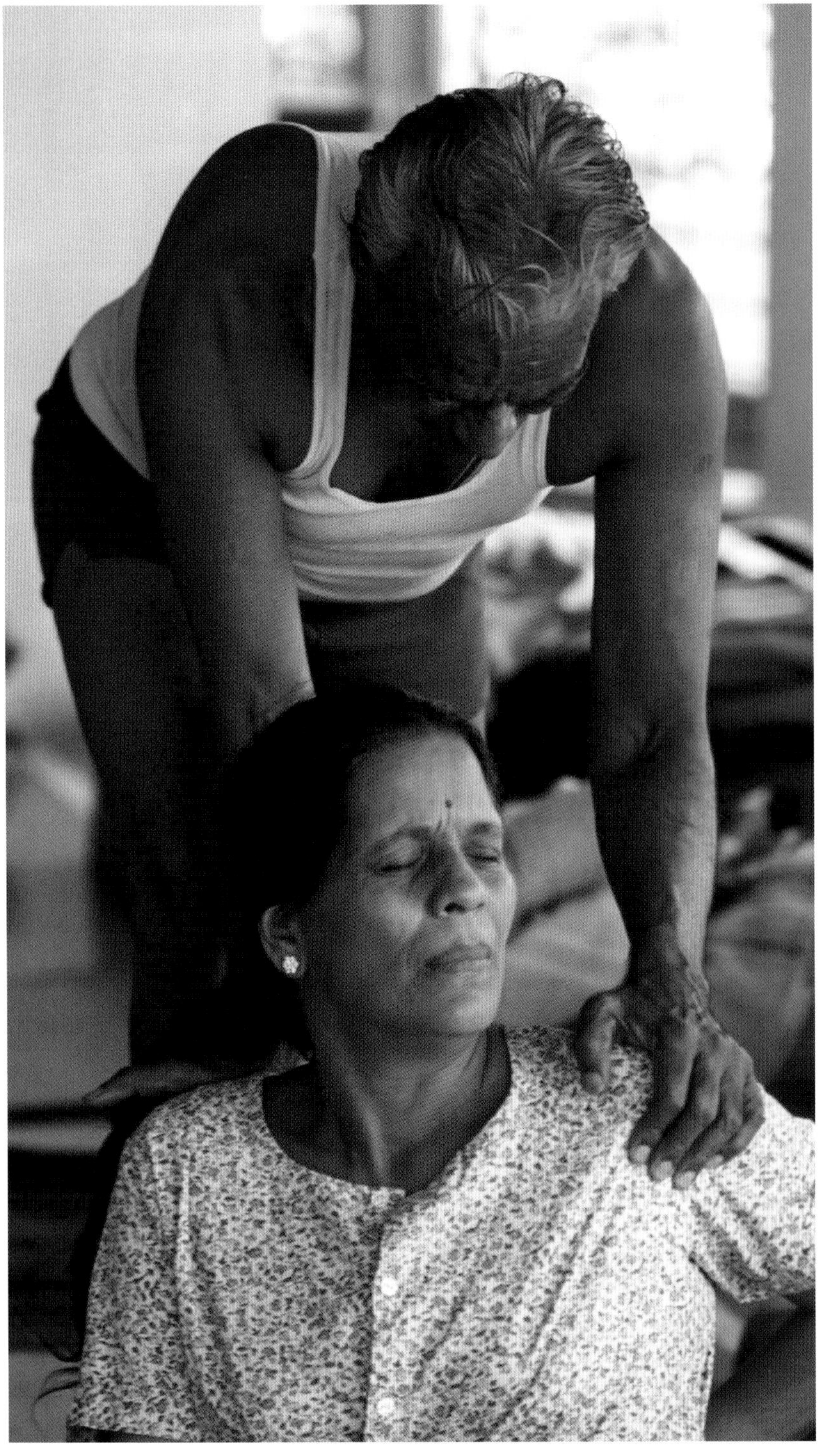

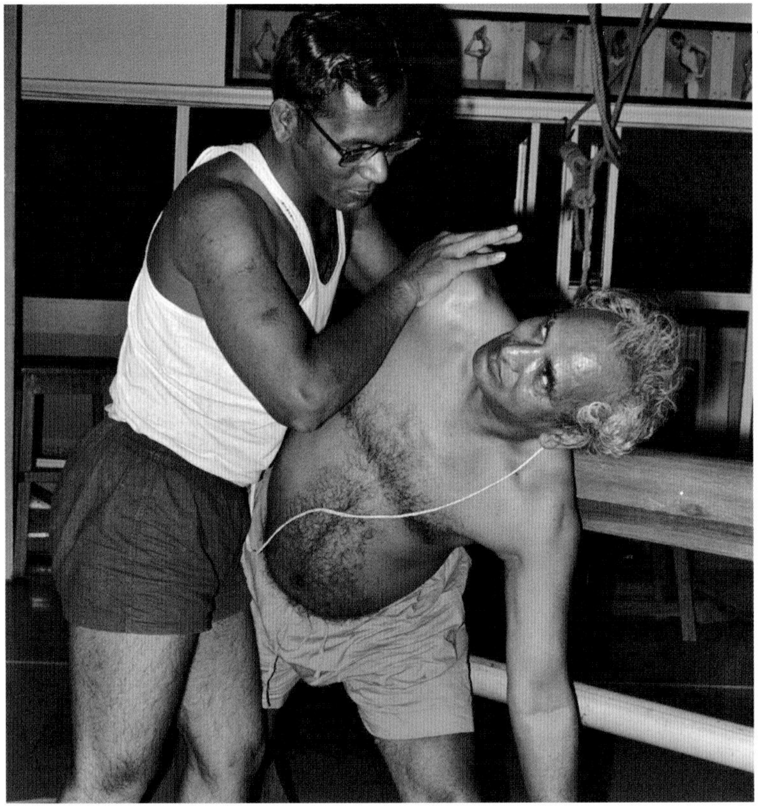

When he was touching the student, how the changes were having the effect in their body. It was fantastic to see. Seeing the person before Guruji helped him and after and I was thinking "What is he doing here?" Slowly, slowly I was learning. When Guruji was in the medical class, while he was holding the rope, which finger was he using? Nobody understood what he was doing. People think he was just holding the rope. No, he was not just holding the rope. He was so sensitive, he was changing the fingers. I saw how when he worked with someone the person changed immediately. It was really marvellous to see.

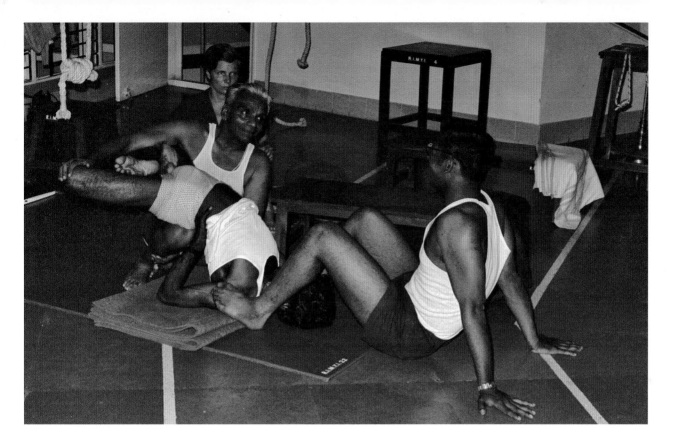

In the class also he was shouting, "Hey, do like this!" and I am looking at him and blinking the eyes and laughing with him. When he is shouting I know he's not angry at all. He is making that person do a little bit more with, "Hey, do this!" But he was not angry at all. This I know exactly. That is why I was often laughing. I'm thinking, "How this man is creating the situation." But sometimes he would tell me with a look not to laugh. Some people thought he was angry in the class, but this was not at all true. He was totally different.

VD

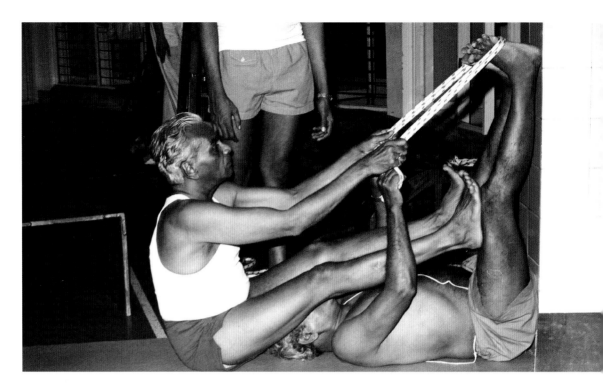

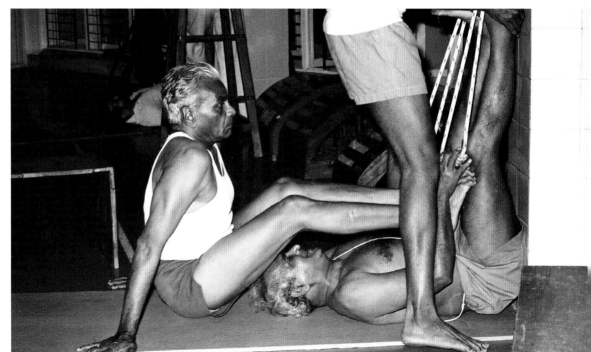

I came across the book, *Iyengar: His Life and Work*. I started doing some *asanas* but it was very difficult to start alone and I also felt bored. After a few months, I met Guruji and that changed my mind totally. I practiced daily with full enthusiasm for hours. My practice became a part of my *sadhana*.

To deepen my practice I visited two Iyengar yoga teachers once a week. I set out on my motor-scooter for the class, but I never reached my destination, as on the journey I crashed into a bus. After two weeks I opened my eyes in hospital. A bus had driven over my right leg and crushed the leg and hip. I had lost a lot of blood by the time I arrived at the hospital and had barely enough haemoglobin to survive.

I was in the hospital for 4 months, undergoing further treatments. Then for 6 months I was at home in the bed on my back. In total I had more than 18 surgeries. Those two years were a mess, with a lot of pain and misery.

I heard people saying that I would never be able to practice again. This also gave me a challenge. I was in touch with Guruji after the accident and he encouraged me so much. He gave me a lot of hope and he asked me not to do anything until everything had healed nicely. Guruji told me that with lots of will power and perseverance, I would be back to my practice. He asked me to go to Pune when I was able to move independently. It took me two years to be able to move and to travel such a long distance by train.

I had been living in pain for a long time and in Pune there was more pain. I also had a lot of fear. Fear of falling, fear of something happening to me. What if something broke again? After the accident I was afraid of everything. He made me do a lot of backward bending *asanas*. One day, I was doing *Viparita Dandasana* on the stool. Guruji came and pushed my chin down with his leg. I was quite suddenly really relaxed and smiling.

What Guruji did was amazing. He knew he first had to remove the fear. At that time the pain persisted and he became quite harsh with me and said "you are living in an ashram and you cannot face this much pain? Can't you accept a little more pain? What is more painful, the accident or what you are doing here?" Guruji showed me how to change. I became more relaxed, more confident and my whole attitude changed. From that time onwards Guruji really started working with me and it was wonderful.

These injuries were many years ago now. The pain, the whole trauma is so far away and I hardly think of it now. Even in my practice I don't think of my injuries. My practice has become my *sadhana* and that gives me inner happiness.

UD (Usha Devi)

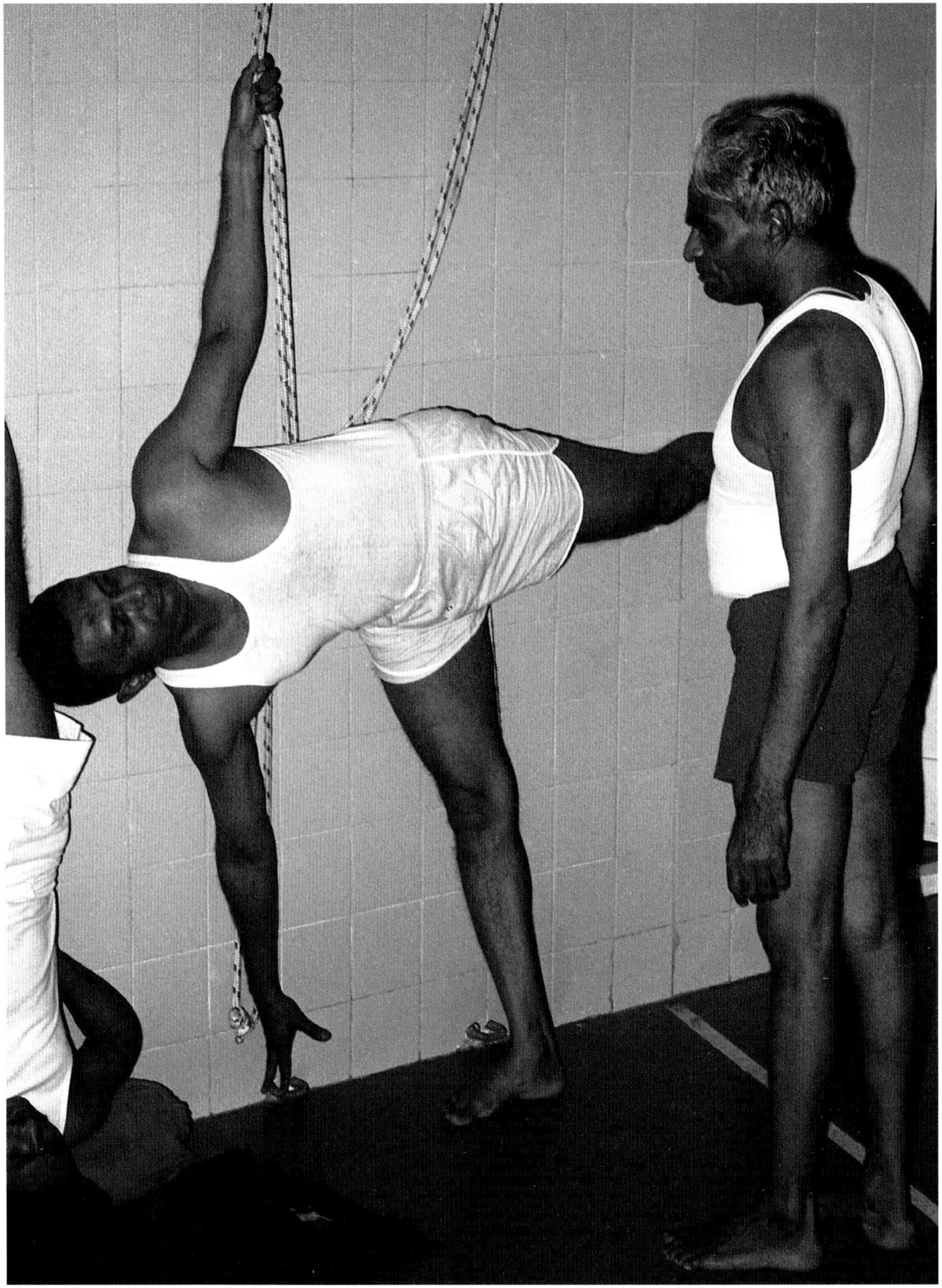

The medical classes were astonishing. There were patients in all kinds of poses, teachers running helter skelter and Guruji walking from one end to the other. There used to be a few teachers constantly helping a specific patient or groups of patients for a few weeks while there would be visitors like us from Mumbai or the foreigners who would be there for a few turns. Guruji moved so fast, adjusting, directing, that it was impossible to keep pace with him. In one of my very early attendances in the medical class, there was a new patient with only one leg as the other had been amputated. Guruji asked me to make him do *Ardha Chandrasana* on the tressler and I happily did it. Guruji watched and did not make any comment so I was happy... it was correct. Then I waited for instructions from Guruji on the next *asana*. Guruji came and said, "What about the other side?" Other side! But, he has only one side. I did not have the courage to ask him, but I wondered how can I make him stand on a leg that does not exist! Guruji then placed a stool below the stump of the amputated leg and made him do *Ardha Chandrasana* on the other side. He then said, "Do you realise how much pain he has on the back where the leg does not exist?" It was something I would never ever have imagined in my wildest of dreams. The student immediately responded with a smile. I never ceased to be amazed—how did Guruji know all this?

RM

Personally what had happened for me was that at one point I had gotten a pinch in the lower back. I didn't realise what was happening and for one whole month I was just struggling and not getting rid of it. My father decided he would tell Guruji that I had this problem. He told Guruji and he said, "Just go and do *Trikonasana* with the back body by the wall." He came to me and grasped my lower arm and then pulled it down. When I came up from the pose, the pain had disappeared, absolutely. I had been struggling for a month or so, he just adjusted it like that, the hand which is down he extended it and pulled it down. He just did that and everything was fine, the pain went away.

BM

163

Guruji had this unique ability to 'see the circuits' within our body. He indeed had X-ray or should I say MRI vision. By looking at the arms and legs, the elbows and the knees—he could assess how the bones, the ligaments, the tendons and cartilage were placed: which side was overworked and which side was underworked. By looking at the shoes of a person, he was able to see which part of the spine was affected. And, after this diagnosis, which happened in milliseconds, he would immediately start on the correction. He corrected with his own hands, his head, his legs and then used the help from his students. I don't think anybody had used yoga effectively as a therapy before him. This entire speciality of yoga therapy has emerged from Guruji's observation and skills. At that time, we were just mesmerised by his ability. But, today I wonder how much he must have studied the human body in the different *asanas* to be able to work so quickly and efficiently.

RM

One time in 1976 when I was in Pune after a particularly bumpy rickshaw ride back to my hotel in Camp, my back started really hurting. During the course of the night I woke up and I felt like I couldn't breathe. My back had gone into spasm and neither I nor my roommate knew what to do. For about two hours I was gasping for breath and around 6 a.m. she got me into a rickshaw and took me to the Institute. We knew that Guruji would be in the practice hall and decided to take a chance that it would be OK.

As she helped me up the stairs, I struggled to breathe, and when we got to the top Guruji was standing there. He took one look at me, didn't say anything and immediately took me to a hanging rope and put me upside down in *Sirsasana*. He told me to clasp my hands together and then he stood with his feet supported by my hands and began to swing back-and-forth. I don't know how long he kept that up but then he physically took me down from the ropes, stood me up at the horse and set me up doing standing poses. I was breathing better but still not quite out of it. He literally put me in those standing poses and worked my body together with the horse until he got me into the position he wanted for each pose. After that he told me to go back to my room and lay down. He said to me, "You will feel like a truck has run over you for 24 hours and after that you will be fine." Twenty-four hours later I was fine and back in the class.

JW

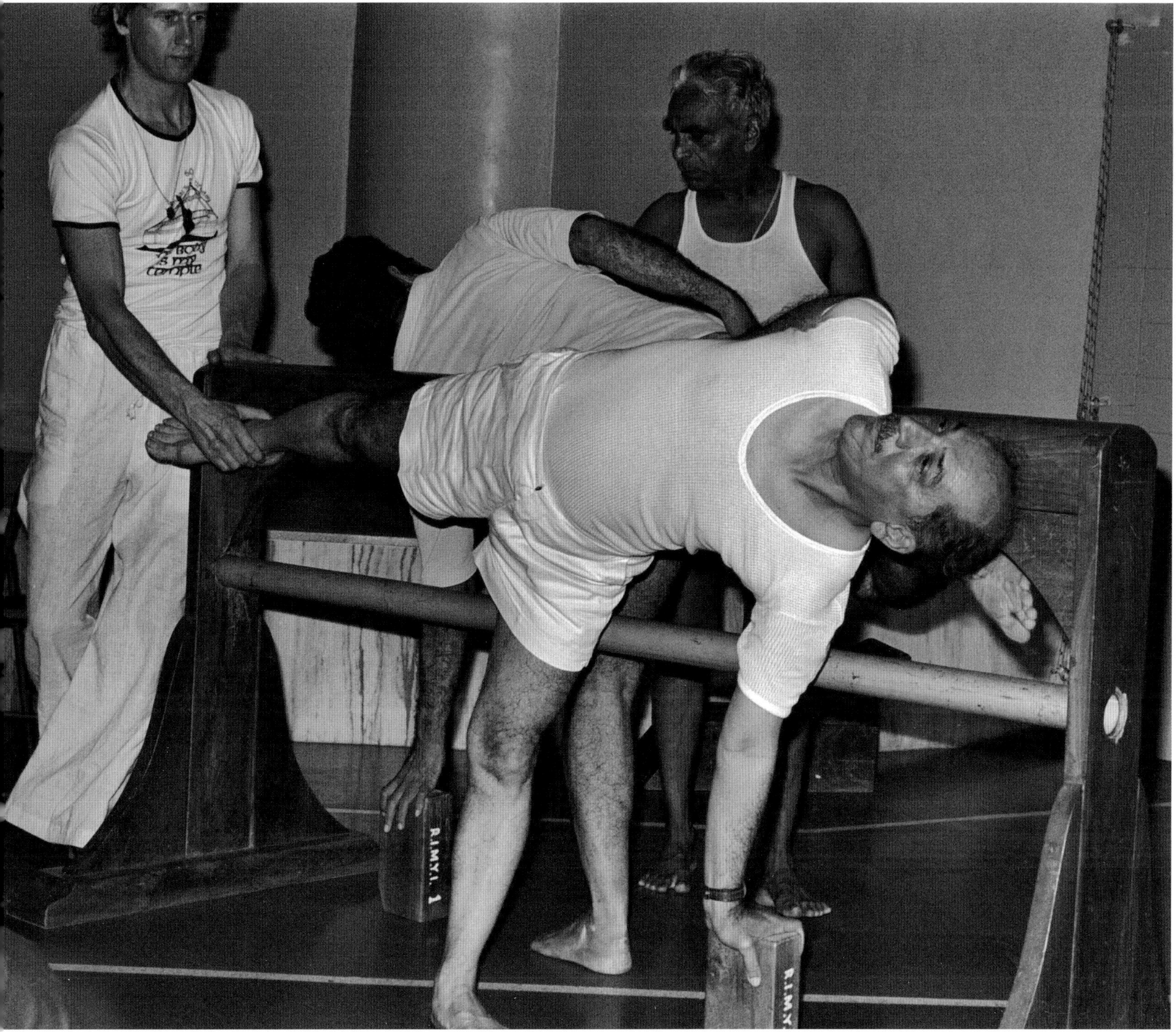
R.I.M.Y.I. 1

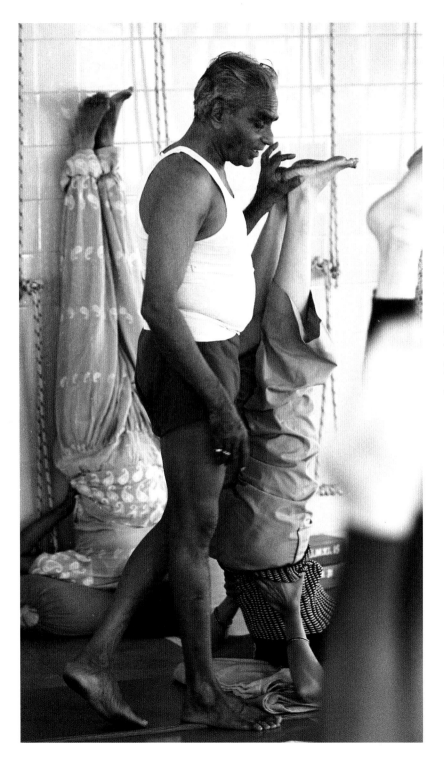

Guruji helped me to reach out to the poorest of the poor in health. The first person that he helped me with was my own father. Guruji gave me a protocol for his heart. My father was given 3 months to live in 1978 unless he underwent a heart bypass operation overseas. Guruji gave us this heart protocol which till today I use for heart patients. And dad lived for 18 more years without surgery.

Guruji was a man who encountered a person suffering on a person-to-person level. I would take patients sometimes to the library at the Institute when he was reading in the afternoon. He would ask me or the person I brought for healing to get into the postures. Sometimes he even walked up to the second floor hall with me and showed me how it had to be done. He's like Mother Teresa—he's an energy within me. So I never let a day go by without an Iyengar practice.

FJP

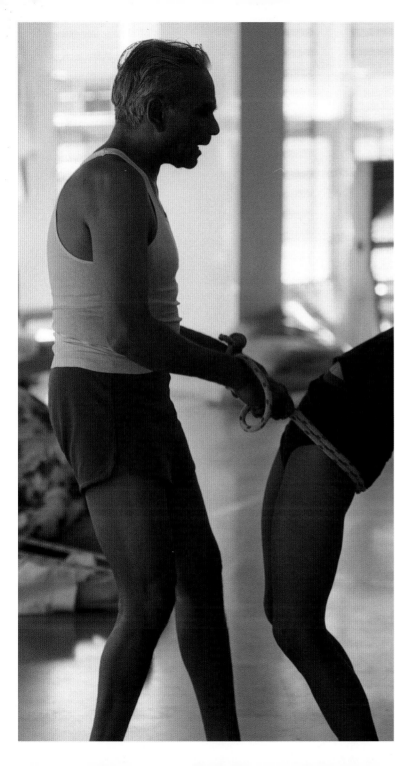

There are very few props in these photos, yet this whole archive catalogues Guruji adjusting students in the *asanas*, propping up students in inversions or holding them for backdrops and guiding them into the pose in the medical classes. Countless people were touched and helped in the classes and their actions and physiognomy were deeply internalised by Guruji. It took years before many of the props were created, and their development and evolution continued thoughout Guruji's life.

ZZ

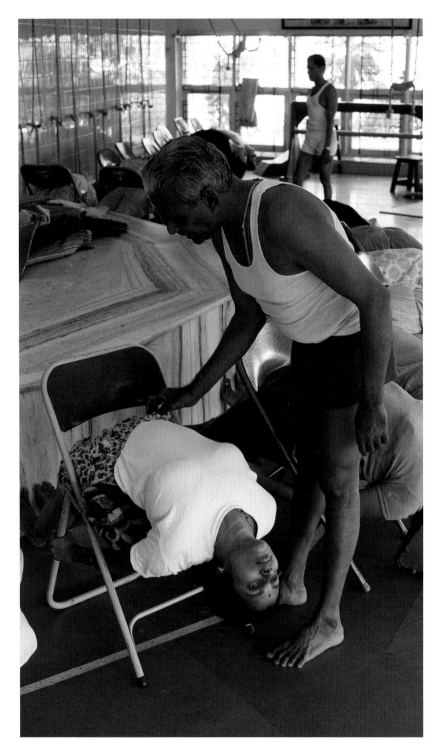

I had fractured two vertebrae in my thoracic spine in a horse riding accident in 1972 and had temporary paralysis. After some time I could do some yoga and was able to have classes with Guruji. I remember in the first class he lined us all up very precisely and put me in the front and centre so he could watch me. He told me I had to do everything and he would watch to see what I could or couldn't do. I had only been introduced to some of the standing poses as I had not been able to participate in classes because of my back. However as he shouted out the names of the poses while quickly demonstrating them, I found myself able to follow along.

During those early classes he watched me, but the one thing I remember best was the day he put everyone on chairs to do backbends. He stood next to me as I went back over the chair. I suddenly felt excruciating pain and dizziness, and I felt a hand immediately pulling me up, and he said,"With pain like that you are not ready to go back yet." and of course he was correct. I felt such caring and compassion from him that I was overwhelmed with emotion. He told me to work hard in standing poses and I did. He constantly checked on me in every pose in those early years to see how I was doing and if I was following. This close attention to what I was doing brought me into a more personal relationship with him and it also made me much more aware of what I was doing. This had a profound effect on my improving, which happened reasonably quickly.

JW

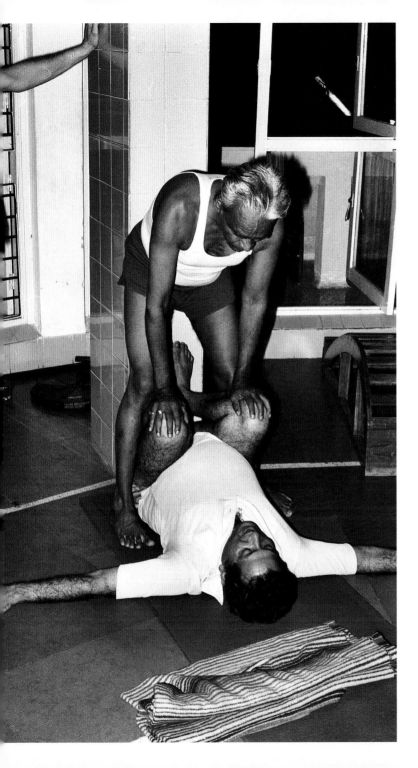

169

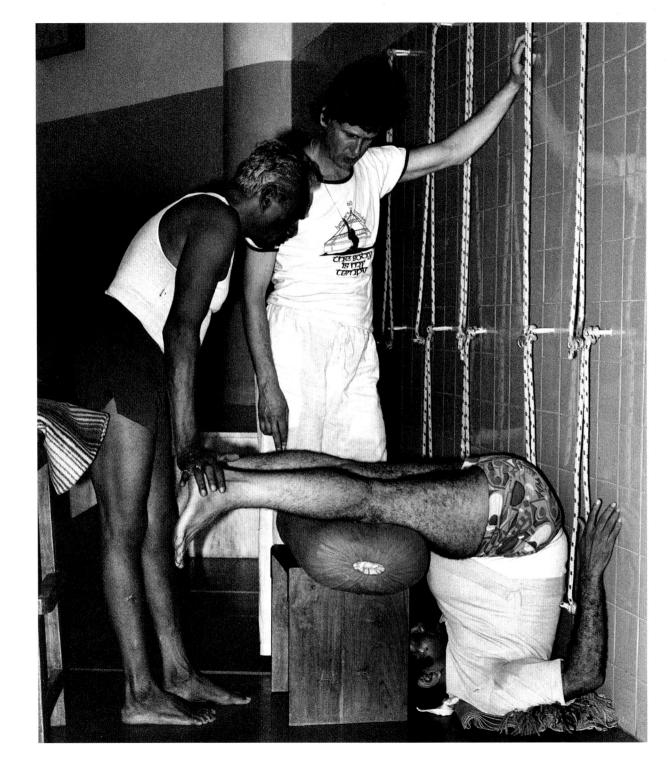

In fact I tried very hard to do exactly what he did and exactly what he said but very, very rarely would he say that it's right. Every so often he would come and correct you in your correction, in your assisting. He would say, "See, this is not how I touch." But we learned a lot. I learned because of that. Every time I would be holding he would say, "That's not how I held." How to hold, how to turn, where to hold, the movement of the skin, the movement of the muscles, the tiny adjustments. It is all those skills that we learned by helping in the therapy classes. The fact was that when he corrected you, you learned it on your own body. For assisting others, that was our ground of training.

His fire was so strong and nothing could escape him. One wrong movement and he would reprimand you. He had amazing energy. I don't know how he managed all those patients—people couldn't walk, people couldn't stand. He would say, "They bring these people only at the last minute when doctors say they can't do anything. Why do you bring them to me?" And then he would turn and walk to the end of the room there. And then he would walk back. Then he would say, "Hey, bring that chair from there or bring that bolster," and then he would start helping them. His compassion! He couldn't turn away anybody. It was amazing to see.

FAR

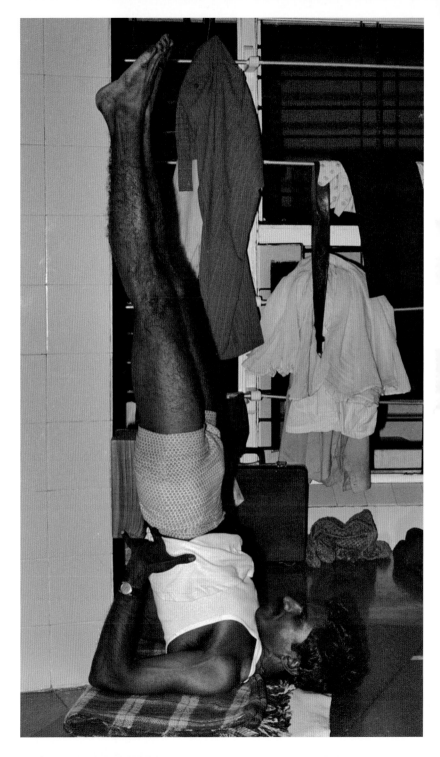

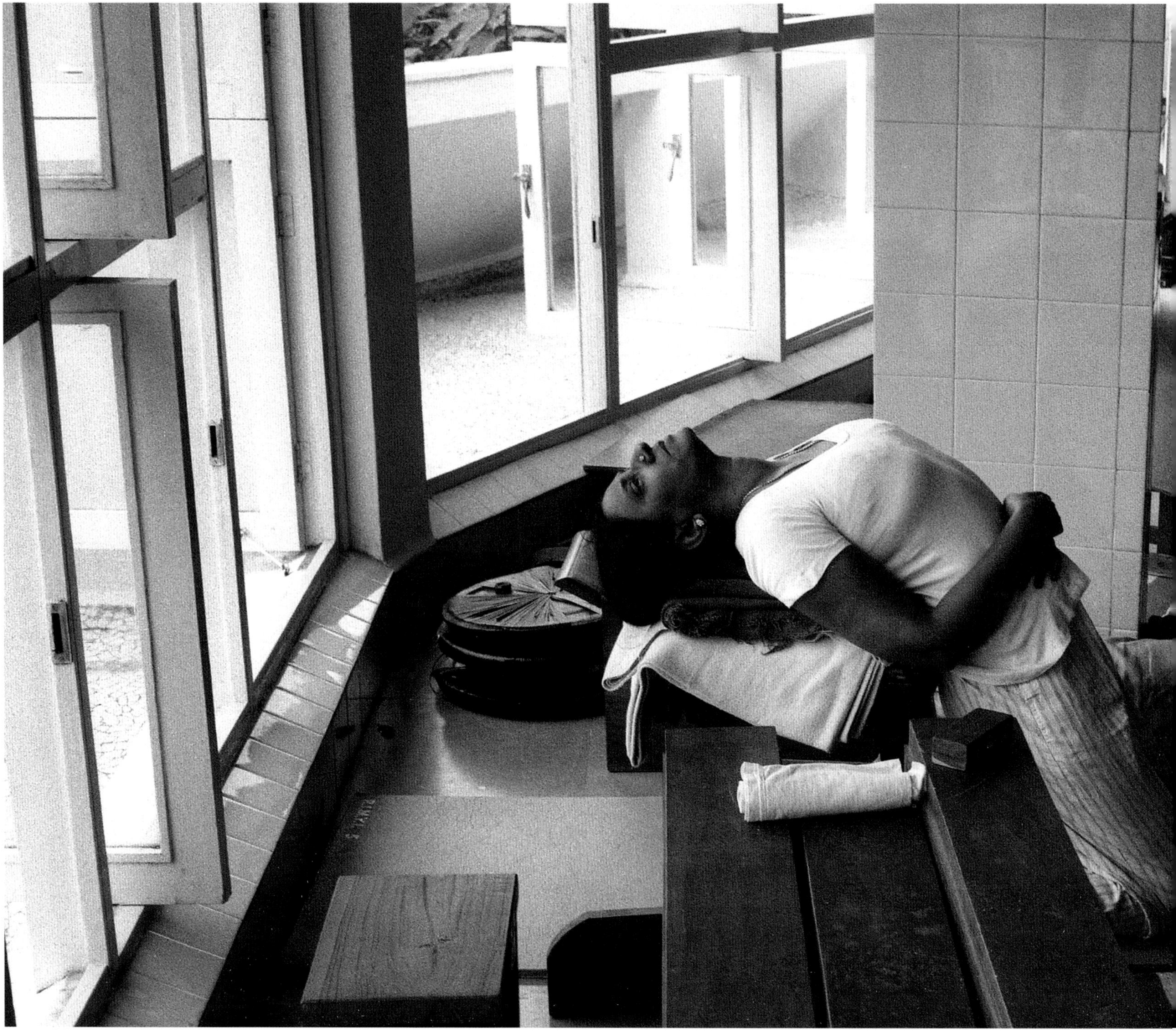

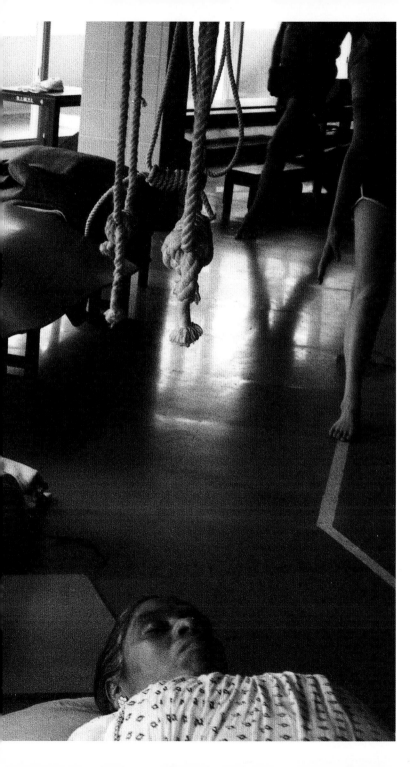

Let's say that Guruji had told me to give a student a certain support/prop. He would say do this way and then help him like that. Then that week is over. Then the next week I see the same person and I might be giving him the same program. Then Guruji used to come from behind and say, "Can't you see that person was different last week. Now he is much better—he can do more." He said, "Don't give the sequencing mechanically. See the person. I have given the sequence for last week, now this person is different which you can see. You have to give them a different sequence." That is how Guruji taught us. Learning like that with Guruji was unbelievable. We were witnessing miracles every day in the medical class.

AJ

The Props

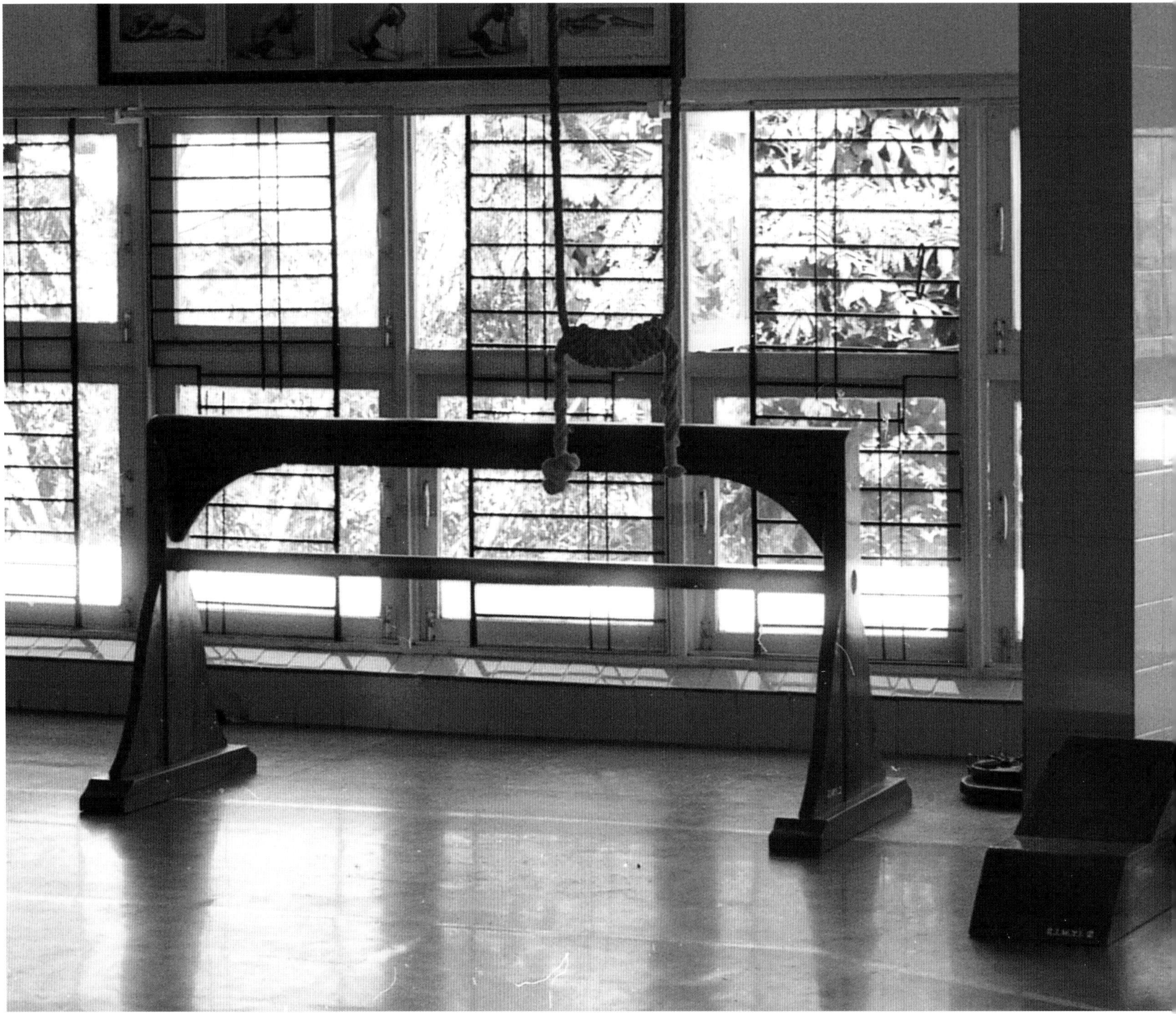

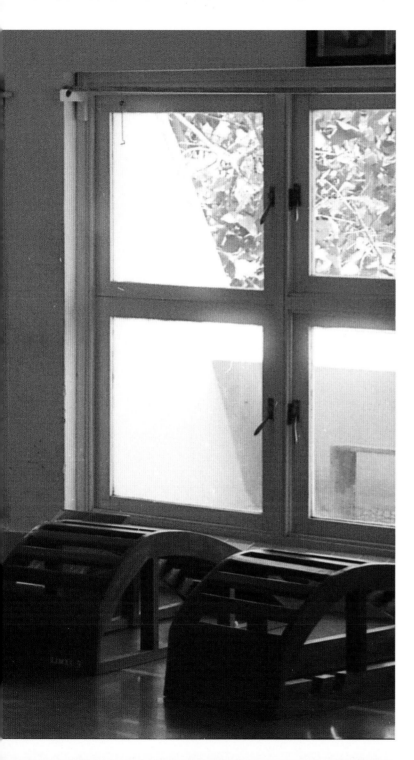

There was only one brick in the whole Institute when Guruji started. The props were invented in front of our eyes.

AJ

I started in Mumbai in 1969 and we only had a single blanket as a prop, even for *Sarvangasana*. Everything was done independently. There were no blocks, no straps, no chairs. I only saw props in 1975 when I came to the Institute in Pune.

JB

He designed in his mind from those early days in the '60s and '70s how the body could be helped to keep a posture and get the benefits of the posture that even a classical practitioner would not get. He would take for instance the way we do *Sirsasana*—he would do it perfectly, but even the best students in our class wouldn't be able to sustain the posture. So I saw him bringing in supports to be able to get the posture so accurately that the benefits would follow.

FJP

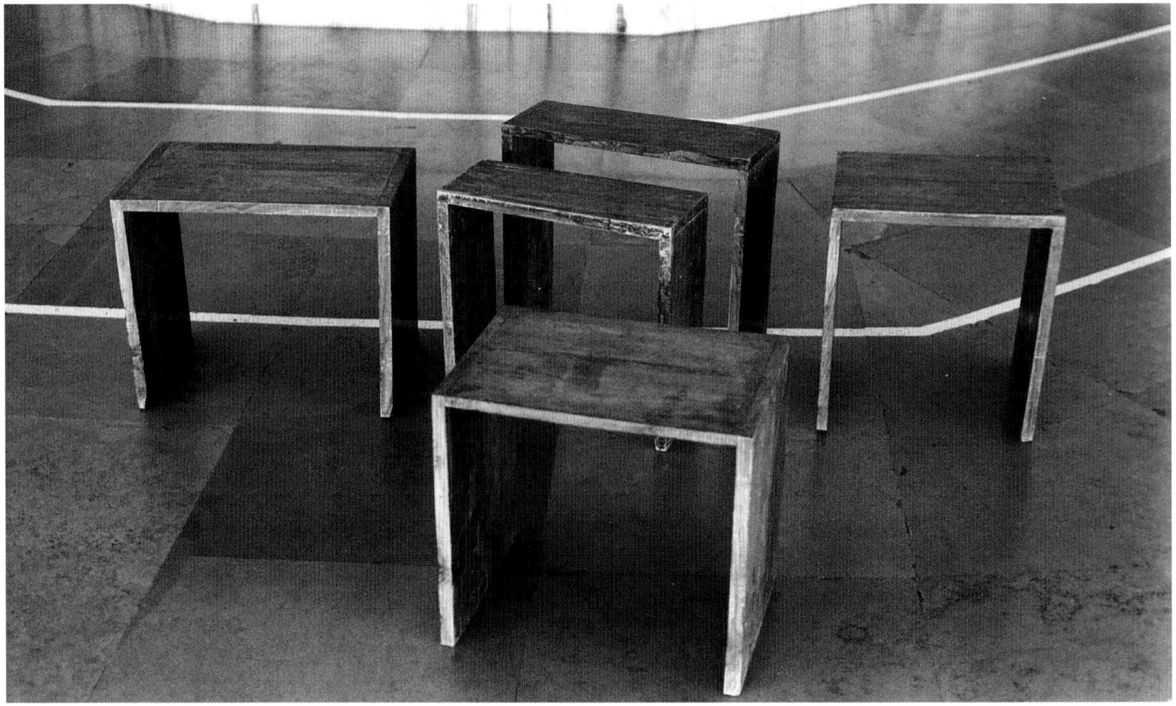

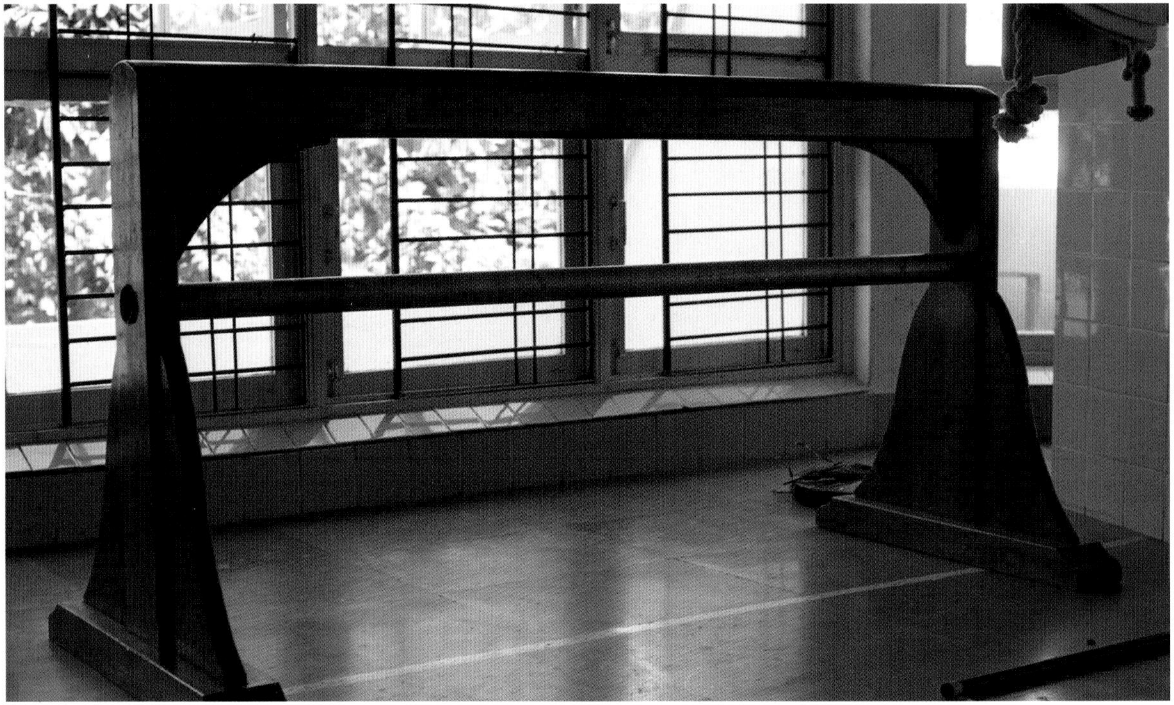

When the Institute opened in 1975, Guruji really started his research into the development of props. The first thing that came was the *Viparita Dandasana* bench. He was thinking and thinking of how to support an older person of 60 or 70 years of age—how can I help him to do the *asanas*, how can I put him in the pose. Guruji was not satisfied with one *Viparita Dandasana* bench and he made some changes. After some time he was satisfied and made different sizes to suit the development of the spines of different students. Guruji was constantly exploring how it works on the different parts of the body. Nobody understands these things—just how much thought of his was behind it.

Next was the *Halasana* box. In the early days, before there were props, if someone needed extra help, Guruji would have them do half *Halasana* either with their feet on the wall or with one of the assistants sitting in front of them and their feet would rest on our shoulders.

There was one *Setu Bandha* bench in the beginning and it was used by some heart patients. These people came after operation or before operation and Guruji would work on how he could open the heart area and then he found the great invention of the *Viparita Karani* box. But it's first use was the extension of the *Setu Bandha* bench. People don't realise this fact.

Back in the '70s one day Guruji had to go to a government office. He was asked to wait for his appointment. While Guruji was waiting there for some time, he saw that right next to him there was a balcony. So he started doing *Trikonasana* holding that balcony bar, then he did *Parivrtta Trikonasana*. From that balcony he got the idea of making the trestler.

Continually the props would develop. Guruji used to come and keep developing the props and ways of helping each individual right up until the end. Guruji was the greatest yoga scientist. Until his death, there was always something new in his mind to do.

PR (Pandurang Rao)

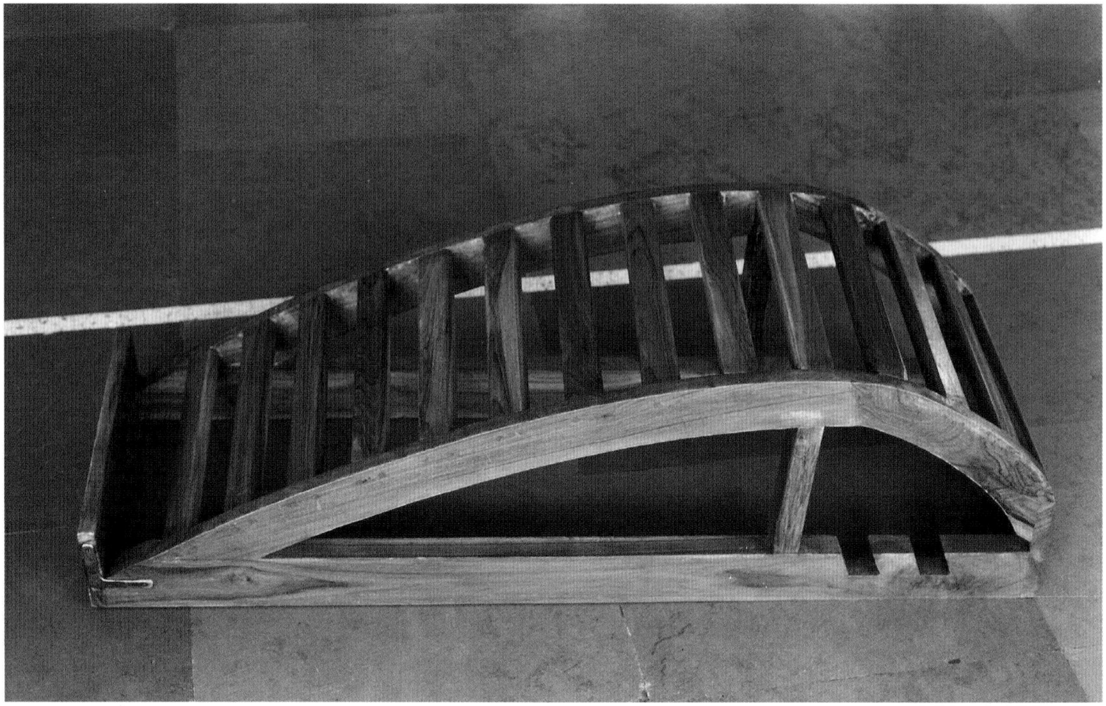

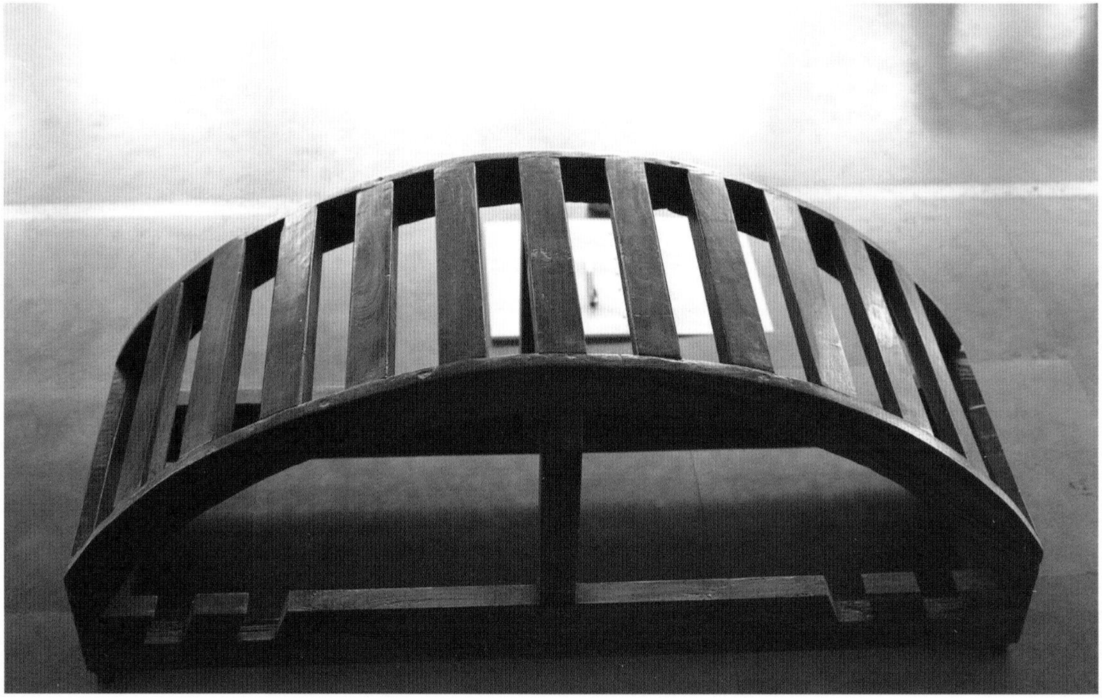

Guruji's yoga props were originally derived from Indian household items such as bolsters, blankets, and window grills. Ropes were positioned on the grills and the *Yoga Karunta* (puppet) was invented. Bricks were literally bricks from building material that Guruji utilised as a yoga prop. Then he developed them into wooden blocks.

Guruji took great care in developing the props for practice. The *Dwi Pada Viparita Dandasana* benches at RIMYI are different in subtle ways. Some open the chest more for the heart while others have a lip at the end to support the feet or additional props. Some do not have a lip. Guruji knew each bench and used them to achieve a particular outcome in the pose.

The *Simhasana* box is sometimes referred to as the heart bench because it is mostly used to support the torso in supine poses. However, it was originally developed exactly for *Simhasana*. To use the box correctly, you lie prone on the upper slant with *Padmasana* legs resting on the lower slant. You can hold the top of the box to lift and lengthen the torso.

One of the last props Guruji created was the *Paschimottanasana* wedge. He told the carpenter what he wanted but he repeatedly sent it back to the carpenter over several months until it was perfected.

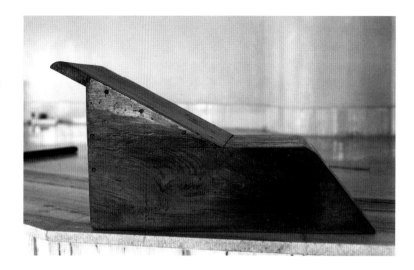

Many Iyengar Yoga practitioners use props to prompt, prod, and promote, whether it be for deep rest or to reach deeper layers of consciousness by going further into a pose than possible without the aid of a prop. The props are not necessarily meant to make one more comfortable; they are often meant to provoke discomfort until the pose becomes effortless.

The props always kept evolving. He was so creative. I learned that a prop is not just for one purpose. He was always inventing new ways of using them from the original one.

LS

Guruji has often made statements about his development of props. I have been there whilst he developed some, a crude rough arrangement that would get developed and refined and further refined. They would have their day. Quite literally, I can remember when Guruji first devised the wedges for knees, for about three months they were getting applied to everyone in the therapy class, behind knees, under backs, beneath shoulders—everyone got to have them in their programme. Quite funny. Once someone gave Guruji a head standing prop, it looks like a toilet seat, but he never employed the prop like that. He actually got a student to sit on it, with their legs wedged in the gap at the front! It seems they needed to compact their knees closer.

Some of the props in these old photos are not in the hall anymore, like the long long *Setu Bandha* benches. Props, or more significantly their usage, comes and goes. There are 'arrangements/adaptations' that get used in the therapy class, but now have disappeared. So too with the props.

It seemed to me that his development of props was like watching the appearance in time of his mind working through the mind-body configuration, studying its secrets, its messages and devising a sculpture around that.

SQ

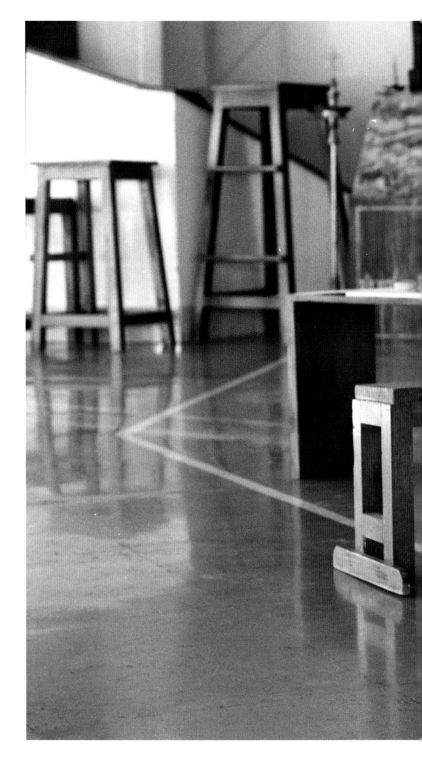

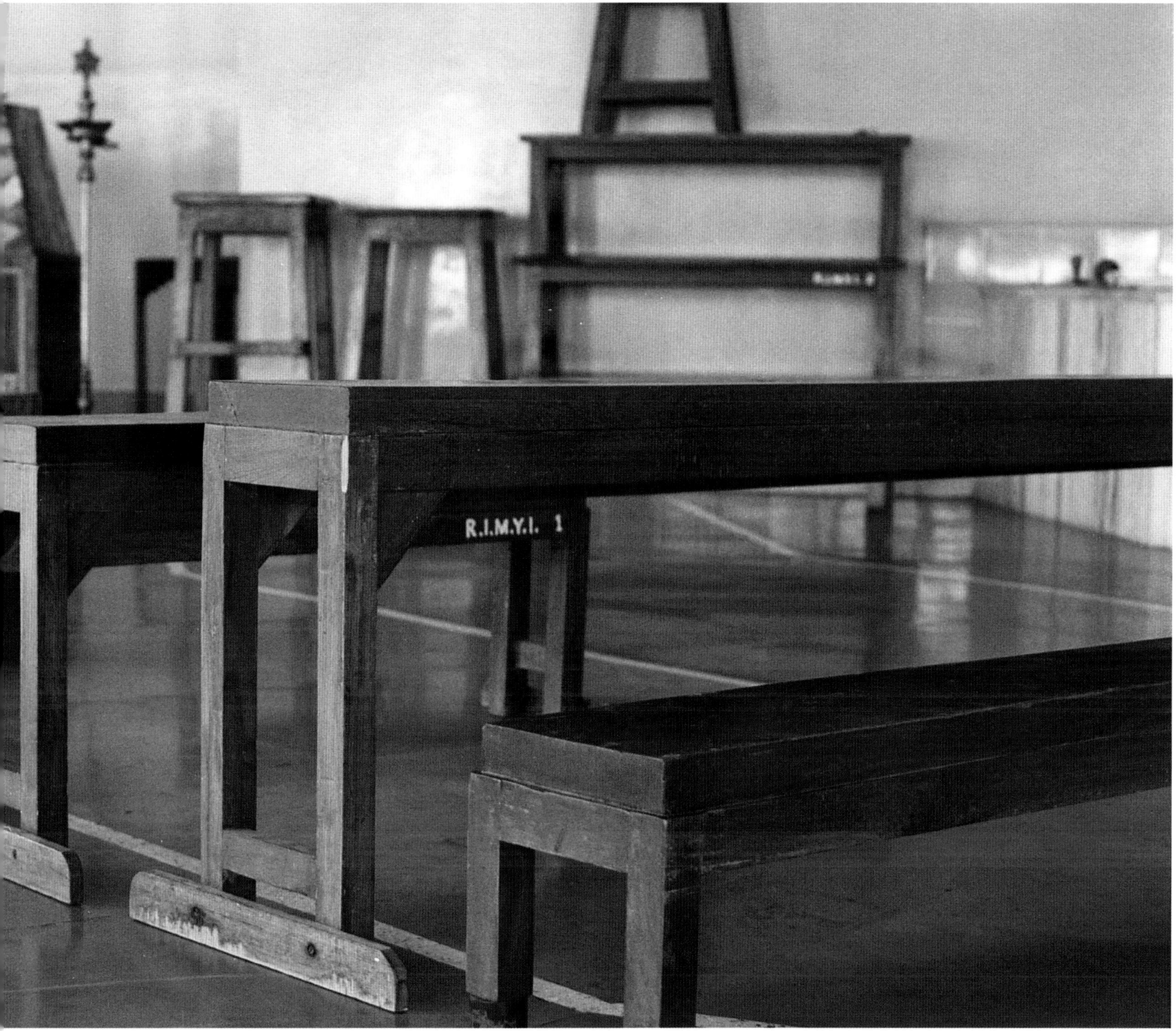
R.I.M.Y.I. 1

Tributes

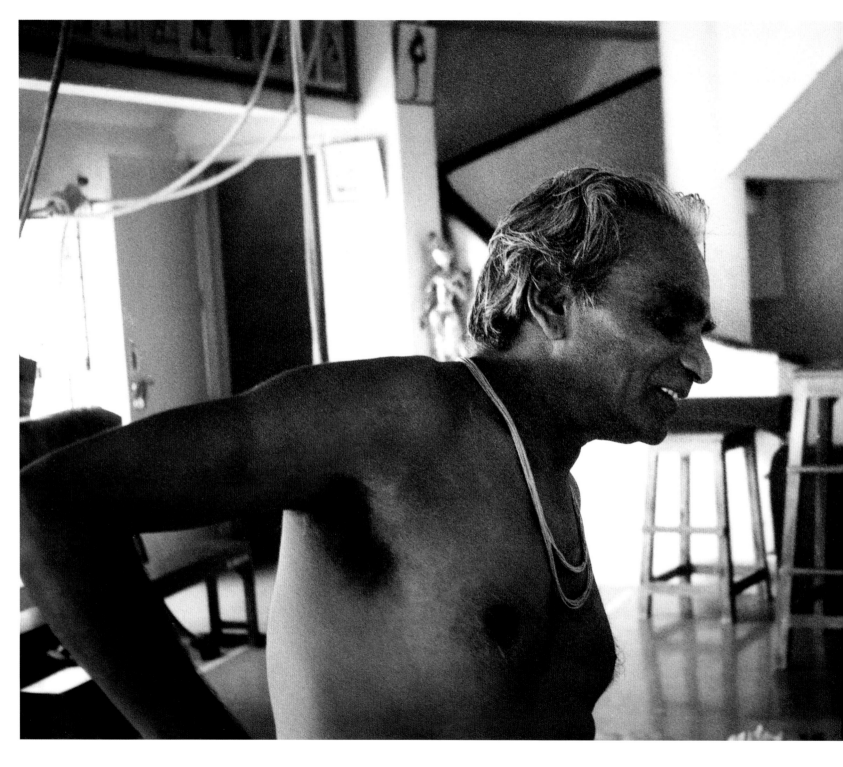

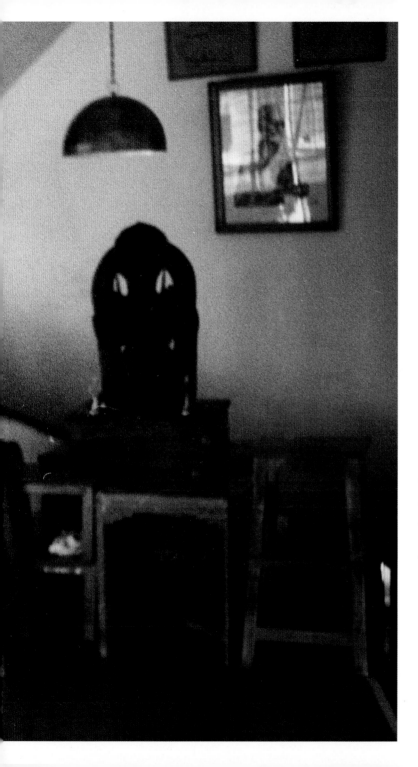

It is indeed a play of destiny that we were born at a time when we could spend so much time with Guruji. We hear, read and talk about enlightened souls but to have been in the presence of one is sure good fortune or past karmas. As time goes by, the impact that Guruji has created on millions of us gets more and more evident. It is so difficult to even comprehend how a single man could revive such a subject and go into such depths and at the same time share with each of us as per our abilities. I am only grateful to God to have been blessed to have such an opportunity.

RM

Guruji was a legend in his lifetime. His teaching is a lifelong challenge to draw out the wisdom latent within the body. No one has shared with us the spirituality of the body as Guruji did!

FJP

The joy and sense of awakening that Guruji taught remain undiminished after 40 years. Is there anything more fulfilling in life? When will we see his like again?

AC

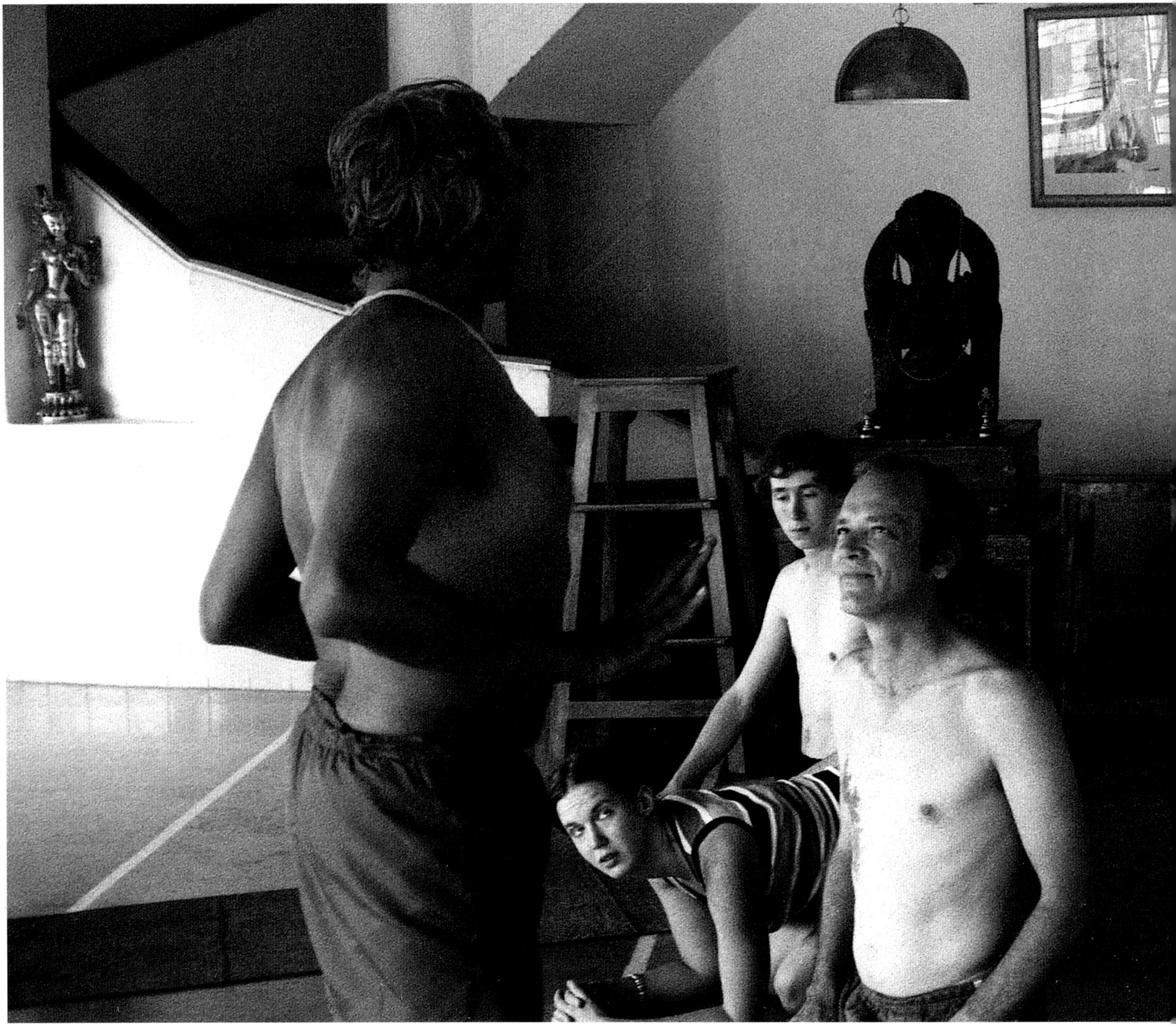

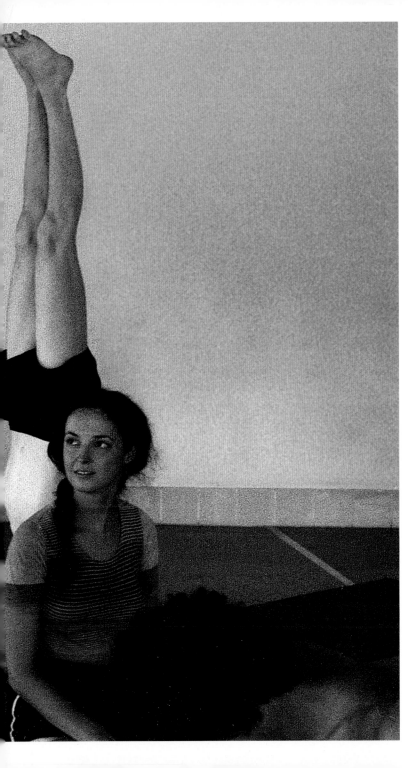

In his presence you had feelings rarely experienced elsewhere; feelings of reverence, admiration and respect. These feelings have never diminished. Your head can understand the meaning of the word guru, but it is your heart that knows and understands the experience of a true Guru, a great spiritual teacher. What a blessing to have Guruji in our lifetime.

KP

Guruji's body was so intelligent, his mind so sharp, his heart so innocent! Just observing his way of being was as much a lesson as receiving his direct teaching.

FB

Guruji was larger than life, fiery and was uncompromising in his teaching. He was also humble, kind and the most generous man I ever met.

BC

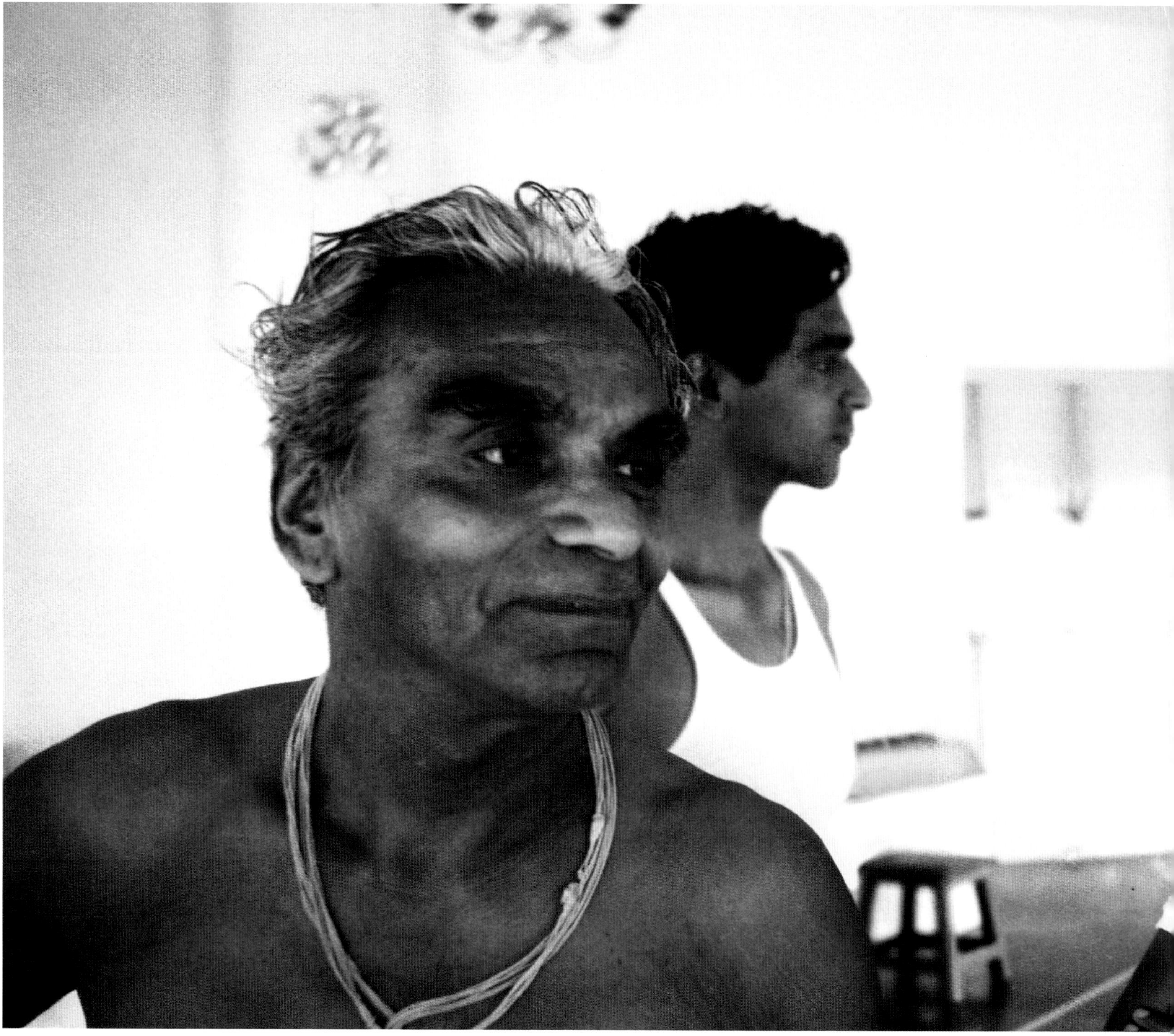

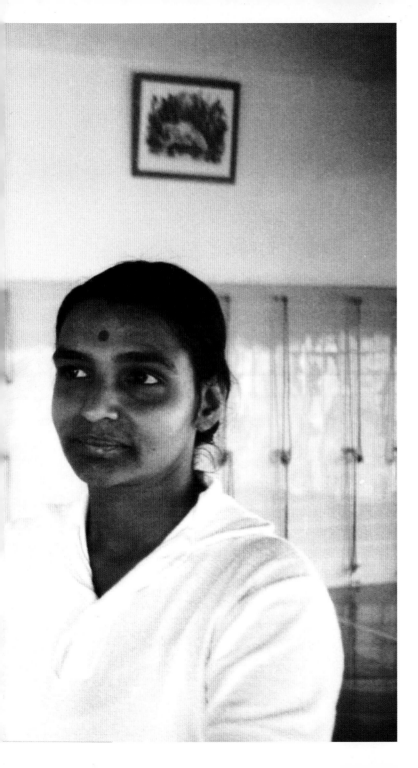

His very presence is what I'm still missing. There is no way that can ever stop. In fact, just closing my eyes or even just thinking of him, I don't need to look at a photograph. Because when I see him there, that's not him. But what I see in my mind, that's him.

FAR

How fortunate were we to live in the time of Iyengar. No words describe the experience or Guruji.

EH

To this day I hear Guruji's voice in every pose. He still helps me reach deep states of absorption.

LS

His presence remains in our hearts, bodies and minds—in our every cell. He permeated our beings and transformed us forever.

PL

He was succinct, brilliant, intense, dedicated. One of a kind, I miss him... Oh, the life and times of Guruji BKS Iyengar!

SC

Acknowledgments

Many people gave help and encouragement to this book project along the way. It would not have come about if Simon Joannou and Hasu Opa Clark had not appreciated the photos and seen their potential when they first saw them. They made the photos available during Abhijata's yoga convention here and there was a big positive response to them. This encouraged me to start the project.

Thanks so much to all of the contributors. Although the photos tell their own story, the contributors really gave life and background to the whole experience at that time in the early days of the Institute.

Special thanks to Lynn Holt who has been living in Pune and studying at RIMYI for many years. She never hesitated to help with transcribing, editing or anything else connected to the project. She was always there with a smile and enthusiasm and gave excellent help and advice. Thanks to my husband Georg Pedersen who took most of the photos. He also loves the book and has been totally supportive in helping it to become a reality. Sarah Burns was very helpful in transcribing and is an excellent editor. Christie Hall also gave invaluable editing advice.

Richard Jonas gave excellent guidance formulating the interview questions. Rajvi Mehta was always helpful in her continuing collaboration, expertise and support.

I am indebted to the Iyengar Yoga Association of Australia for their financial help that enabled me to have Priyadarshi (PD) Sharma do the graphic design and layout. He was a pleasure to work with and did an excellent job. Special thanks to the Presidents of the Association, Simon Joannou and Darrin McNally who recognised the value of the work and helped to get the grant.

I was in Pune at RIMYI recently and was greatly encouraged with the project after showing it to members of Guruji's family who liked how the initial rough draft was proceeding. I was especially impressed by Sunitaji's enthusiasm for the book. That meant a lot to me and I felt I must be going in the right direction. Many thanks, as always, to the whole family of Guruji BKS Iyengar and especially to Geetaji for her interest and encouragement in the project for the last few years.

Julia Pedersen